Everybody Wants to Go to Heaven,

Just Not NOW!

A Practical Guide for
Assisting Others
During Their Last
Days of Life

Pati Hope

EVOLVE TO LIVE,
PUBLISHING DIVISION

ISBN: 978-1-4507-4600-7

Cover and interior design by Tabitha Lahr
Front cover photo: oak tree set against blue sky
© Marilyn Barbone/www.123rf.com
Back cover photo: Ruby-throated hummingbird
© Steve Byland/www.123rf.com

Printed in the United States of America

Dearest Sisters,

It's been my pleasure. I'm looking forward to meet you All! I'm looking forward to many years of friendship! Thank you for the work you do! My wish for you, that you find some words of comfort from my life's experiences!

May God Continue to bless you & your work ♥ Pati

We're all in bodies that are going to die,
but we act as though they're not.

We don't die, other people do. Death is not the end of life,
it is simply an aspect of life. Life flows on ceaselessly.

~ Carlos Castaneda

DEDICATION

With love and gratitude I dedicate this book to my Pop. It is because of his courage to participate fully in his life, all the way until his last breath, that his family was able to experience the incredible spiritual journey one takes as they begin the process of leaving the body behind.

And to my friend Hannah, who patiently listened (a captive audience) as I read her my stories and then anxiously waited for her verdict. The first day we spoke of dying as simply a transition of the soul, she said to me, "When you're dead, you're dead and that's that!" And yet, she didn't really believe it because twenty years earlier, she had etched on the family tombstone in Irish:

Ni crioch ach athfhas

Meaning: It's not an end; it's a new beginning!

CONTENTS

PART 2.

Being Present with Those in Transition

INTRODUCTION

My dad's passing was a process that my four adult children were very much involved with. After his transition, I wanted to send each of them a card, give them some sort of explanation or words of comfort around what had happened to their Papa. I wanted them to see the beauty of the *crossing over* experience rather than the upsetting, or even spooky connotation that I had always associated with dying.

When I brought my mother home from the hospital for her final days on this earth, my then teenage boys fled to their rooms and barely came out—not even to eat! They were older when my dad passed, and had been living with him in his house at the time of his illness. My dad was alert until his final breath, which helped take the mystery out of his dying.

Over the years, I've spent time with many people at the end of their lives, and I've come to see that what we call *life* isn't just about this life at all! It's about the evolution of the soul. This life is what the soul uses to help it evolve to Oneness with God. It became clearer to me that we truly are spirits, here in bodies, for the short period of time that we are on this earth. It is true, our bodies will die, but our spirits will continue to live, forever! They never die.

As I witnessed people's dying processes, there seemed to be three lessons that everyone that I had been with at the end of their life all had in common. Everyone had to learn to let go, receive, and to trust not only themselves, but also God.

We live in a very exciting time to be finished with our walk on this earth. We live in a time when many books have been written and incidents have been shared about near-death experiences. Countless souls who have had these experiences have come back to share with us their understanding, often with the same excitement as one might anticipate the birth of a child, or as a child might look forward to Christmas, so that we too may know.

> *Death isn't something to be feared, but something to look forward to!*

As I have gotten older and experienced the crossing over of others, death no longer frightens me the way it did when I was younger. In fact, I have come to see dying as not only a very spiritual experience, but also as the end of this frontier that we know as life. We have mastered what we needed to learn on earth, and now we find ourselves at the edge of the next frontier—life after death: the continuation of the soul's journey, not the end of it.

I feel that it is not only a privilege but also an honor to be present with those in transition. Leaving the body behind, which frees the soul, is an extremely holy time.

I certainly don't want to make light of the fact that dying is still a funky phenomenon for many of us, especially those who are young or who haven't experienced it before. My illumination has come from life experiences, reading, and people who have mysteriously crossed my path at one time or another, sharing with me their insights, for which I am forever indebted.

This little book simply contains the things I have learned and things that have helped me to see that leaving this earth is just part of the whole journey of the soul.

It is my hope that it will be a tool that may help to bring some peace to the ones who are journeying home and some comfort for those left behind.

> *Dying is part of the process of living.*
> *Every **body** is born, every **body** dies;*
> *the spirit lives forever!*

MANY RELIGIONS ~ ONE TRUTH

Through the search to find myself, I had the opportunity to learn from many different spiritual traditions. I found it hard to believe that God would use only one way to reveal Himself and connect with His people.

A nun explained it to me this way: "It's like going downtown. There are many roads that lead to downtown, but there is still only one downtown." So it is with God. There is one God, but there are many different names used for God. Regardless what you believe, there's still just one Creator. There are many ways to connect with our Creator, many different faith traditions, but still one Supreme Being. Thus, spirituality became a forerunner in my quest to find my purpose in life. Searching different spiritual traditions for truths I could call my own opened my mind, heart, and spirit.

According to Elisabeth Kübler-Ross, "Spirituality is the awareness that there is something far greater than we are, something that created this universe, created life, and that we are an authentic, important, significant part of it and can contribute to its evolution."

I was speaking with a priest friend of mine, who is also a professor in theology, about a type of meditation. When I commented, "That is the same teaching of the Native American Spiritual Tradition," he replied,

"Of course, the *Truths* are all the same."
And to that I add, **"Love is the common denominator."**

There are many religions because there are many different kinds of people. Each religion speaks to a certain individual according to his or her life experiences. Religion simply becomes a place where like-minded people can come together, but there is only one Truth, one God, one Creator, one Higher Power. Use whatever name brings you comfort, a God of your own understanding.

Don't get hung up on the language I use in this book. The words are flexible. Change the language to make it your own. Notice any resistance without judgment.

I've tried to examine the differences between the words *spirit* and *soul* through spiritual resources and in the dictionary. The only thing I have come up with that explains the difference is from Master Li, founder of the *International Sheng Zhen Society*, who states, "The soul is the vehicle of the spirit on this realm." That said, I use the words spirit and soul interchangeably.

Part 1

Understanding Our
Purpose on Earth and
the Process of Our
Final Transition

Chapter 1

WHY WAIT?

The day before my dad crossed over into his new life, I walked into his bedroom to find him sitting in the blue rocking chair beside his bed. As I went to say good morning, he blurted out, "Waiting to die is bullshit!" I had to laugh and answered, "Well, I'll have to agree with you on that one, Pop!" (One of the few things we ever agreed on!)

However, his words gave me food for thought. Really, waiting to die should be a time filled with grace, a time of preparation, and a time of resting. Like the anticipation before any journey, it's a time of gathering information and getting things ready to leave.

My dad was very lucky in the fact that I had already experienced my mom's (and several others') crossing over, so I was better prepared to assist him. We read books

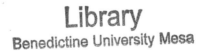

about what to expect, like *Life After Death* and *Embraced by the Light*. We read Bible verses and played meaningful songs. I listened as he reminisced, made him his favorite foods, and was able to just be present for him. We talked about the other experiences I'd had with others leaving their bodies and what to expect as the time drew nearer for his soul to move on.

My experience has been that part of the lessons of this life's journey, for everyone I've been with, is learning to let go, trust and receive. That proved to be true for my dad as well. My dad had to let go of his "stuff" making the trip from his home in rural Missouri to California (letting go) and then let his family care for him (learning to receive). He never wanted to be a burden, as he put it, but in the end he had the courage to say *yes!* (trusting.) He was able to talk about his life, his regrets, his accomplishments, what he never understood, and what he never got to finish.

My dad and I had time together to clear up some of our own issues, and for my family it was an opportunity to show their love, to give of themselves, and to come to terms with his leaving.

I admire my dad. When it's time for my journey home, I hope I am as brave as he was, and that I'm able to say *no* to the extraordinary measures we sometimes use to keep ourselves alive. Why do we do this to ourselves? Are we afraid to let go? Are we afraid of the unknown?

*Do not be afraid of death. It does not exist.
You have to keep a very open channel, an
open mind and no fear. Great insight and
revelations will come to you. You don't
have to do anything except learn to get in
touch, in silence; within yourself...there
are no coincidences.*

~ Eliszabeth Kübler-Ross

*Trust that everything is orchestrated for
your highest good!*

THE PURPOSE BEHIND THE WAITING

Before we can begin to embrace, comprehend, and fully understand the process of dying—a simple letting go of the vehicle (body) that is used to house the spirit/soul in this life—maybe we need a glimpse into why we are here on this earth in the first place.

Over and over again, it has been revealed to me that the ultimate purpose for the soul in this earthly life is to learn how to love—unconditional love, for the things in this world and for others. But the hardest and most important thing is to learn to love ourselves. We cannot give what we don't have; we cannot offer what we don't know. Now, while we all need to learn about love and how to love, I also believe that each soul has a different path to walk, with different things to learn along the way. This is one of the reasons that judging the life of another is pointless. The trials in this life are simply to help our souls to learn the lessons they have come to learn. These lessons are the fuel, so to speak, used to help propel the soul forward after we leave the body behind for all eternity.

The journey of my soul is mine. Learning how and what I am here to learn requires that I follow my own heart and not just live or conform to a family code or a culture because it's familiar. I am learning to be honest and authentic in all relationships—the relationship with myself first, and then with others, including God.

So what is the purpose of this time of waiting? It's simply an opportunity, a gift if you will! When we found out that my mother had cancer of the throat, someone from church said, "Cancer is a gift from God!" *Yeah right,* I thought, *I suppose it's a gift if you're not the one who has it!* But later I would find out that it truly was a gift—a gift of time. It was a time to get her affairs in order and a time to say goodbye.

> *We must simply BE in our unknowing as we wait to know. It is a time of asking for what we need, trusting that, even as we wait, it is given. These times demand a naked vulnerability and a discipline of patience. As we await inspiration, perceived as apparent inactivity, there is a generative process.*
>
> ~ Doris Klein, CSA, Heatbeats Card Series

Waiting, by definition, is a period of pause. And for anyone who's studied music, you know that it's the pauses between the notes that create the music. It's the stopping, resting, and waiting among the notes that make a symphony beautiful to experience.

Other synonyms for waiting include *preparing* and *reflecting*. *Preparing* means to put things or oneself into readiness; to get ready. *Reflection*, as defined by Mr. Webster, is "a time of careful consideration." The word *reflect* is the best of all. Like a mirror; *to reflect* is "to be turned or cast back as light." So, in the waiting there seems to be the invitation and the opportunity for a period of pausing, and still again I ask, *why wait?* May I suggest that it is in this pausing that we've been given a special gift of time to ready ourselves for what's ahead with thoughtful and careful consideration? It's a time for getting our inward and outward affairs in order, a time for saying things that were never said, for hearing things that were never heard, and a time to let go, receive, and trust.

In many Christian faith traditions, the period of Lent lasts forty days—forty days of waiting, for preparing inwardly for the resurrection of Jesus. Then there's Advent, the four weeks before Christmas, which again is time set aside to wait and remember the birth of baby Jesus.

This waiting, in preparation for something wonderful to happen, reminds me of the birth of my children. It was a time of preparing the nursery, reading, practicing, and anticipating, as well as listening to others share their stories of what to expect. It was a time to understand the birthing process so that I was able to participate in my children's births to the fullest extent possible. Childbirth is not something that happens to us, something that we have no control over, but rather something we should participate in completely. For me, childbirth was an experience I looked forward to because I had prepared for it. It was not something to be feared due to lack of knowledge or understanding. In fact, knowledge is power.

I grew up in a house where we weren't encouraged to think or were not even allowed to ask questions. "Just do as your're told," was the motto in my family. But as I've evolved personally, I see the problems with that theory of living. It gives someone else, whether it be religious figures, doctors, lawyers, etc., a place on a pedestal, when in fact the trust should be accepted within ourselves first. I think we should be encouraged to go out and to seek knowledge from the *experts,* but then to make our conclusions for ourselves, rather than to rely on others. When we understand things, we can begin to embrace and then we can easily move with them.

Let's go back to the word *reflection* for a moment. *Reflection* is the result of pause and preparation. Once again, the word *reflect* refers to being *turned or cast back as light.* So, through this personal time of pausing, resting, and preparing ourselves for what's to come, we become the Light. We actually begin reflecting back to others what's happening within ourselves, what we're experiencing not only outwardly but also inwardly. By allowing others to be a part of and a witness to our lives all the way until we breathe our final breath on this earth, we give them the opportunity and honor to experience this Light.

It appears that this *waiting* is an important time in a person's life on many levels. Why would it be any different in the preparation of the soul leaving the body?

My experience has been that the natural slowing down of our bodies and minds helps this time of reflection along. If we continue to perform as we used to when we were younger—constantly moving, constantly doing—we will not be able to listen or pay attention to the transitioning. What if the final lessons are not yours alone, or even yours at all?

The *waiting* seems to have a purpose with possibilities of truly being a gift not only for ourselves but also for those who assist, witness, and spend time waiting with us, pausing, preparing, and reflecting.

MY DAD'S DECISION TO *WAIT*

My dad was living in Missouri at the onset of his illness, and most of his family was living in California. He was diagnosed with renal failure and opted not to go on dialysis. When I arrived for a weeklong visit, I found that he was already using his oxygen full-time, throwing up frequently, and feeling miserable.

One morning my dad announced that he had nearly "checked out" the previous night. I knew my dad, and I knew what he meant when he said *checked out!* "How were you planning to do it?" I asked. My dad was a gun collector and he pointed his finger to his temple. "Wow," I calmly replied. "I totally respect how you want to live and leave this world, but I'm not cleaning up that mess, so you'd better think of another way!" He said nothing, and I continued. "Pop, what if the lessons you're meant to learn from this life come at the moment of your last breath on this earth? What if they're not your lessons at all? What if they're for the rest of us? Will you take that away because of your fear?"

Well, I'm happy to say that he chose to stay and that we all received lessons, including him, because of his courage and willingness to participate fully in the *leaving of his body*. We all learned and loved more than we possibly could have otherwise.

My dad finally agreed to leave his home in Missouri and travel with me to California where he spent his final six weeks on this earth. He had been a wise investor and owned property in the town I was living in. My two adult boys moved into his house with him so he had company in the evenings, and I came in the mornings for the day shift. We were all able to experience his crossing over to the next world fully because of his willingness to move through his fear.

Chapter 2

WHY ARE WE HERE ON THIS EARTH?

Life is full of transitions. I believe that we are in constant transition from the moment we inhale our first breath when we enter into this life, until we exhale our last breath when we leave, and throughout every moment in between.

In fact, did you know that we lose between thirty and forty thousand dead skin cells every minute of each day? That is nine pounds of dead skin cells we loose each year! We are constantly in transition, constantly changing, learning, and evolving.

Back when I was resisting life changes that had come my way, my spiritual director told me that we are on this earth to learn, and that if I continually had my brakes on, using every bit of energy that I had in order to be sure things remained, "as they always had been," then I was wasting my time here on this earth. The energy I was using to resist was the same energy I could be using to move forward.

Now, I have come to understand that we are here on this earth for the evolution of our souls. From my research and experiences, I've discovered that life is about learning to love. Learning how to love others and the things around us, of course, but I've found out that often the hardest is to learn to love ourselves. Next, the mission of our soul is to acquire other lessons and knowledge that we as individuals choose to learn for the purpose of helping our souls to move forward toward heaven and oneness with God, for all eternity.

> *Before I formed you in the womb I knew you*
> *and before you were born I consecrated you . . .*
> ~ Jeremiah 1:5

Further, I believe that at times, we co-create with God by choosing what kind of lessons we'll learn, who will come into our lives to help us learn them, and what kind of body we'll use as a vehicle to house our souls in this life. I use to like talking about the Journey of the Soul as a horizontal, linear progression because it helped me to visually see that we are moving forward through life. However, in writing this book, I saw that the soul's journey is truly vertical in nature, ascending upward toward Heaven and Oneness with God. Then it occurred to me that, really, it's like the Christian Cross. It's about both: the horizontal, life and relationship with others, as well as vertical, our connection with the Divine. The Journey of the Soul diagram helps to illustrate my point.

Only the body dies, the spirit lives forever!

The Journey of the Soul

Why are we here on earth? It's simply about the Journey of the Soul.

IT'S ABOUT ETERNITY!

We've come to earth to learn how to *love* and to learn other lessons that will help to propel our soul upward, towards Oneness with God.

Once we drop the body, we continue to evolve, attaining oneness with God and heaven.

Birth ~ Acquiring a vehicle to house the soul while here on earth.

Body ~ The vehicle used by the soul while on this earth.

Soul ~ Lives forever.

Life ~ Learning lessons on earth to help propel the soul upward.

Death ~ "Crossing over" is simply leaving the body behind. The soul continues its journey toward oneness with God and heaven.

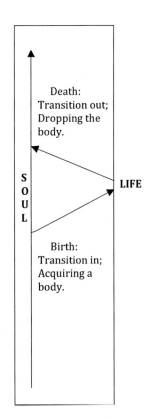

Chapter 3

HOW DO OUR SOULS EVOLVE?

"[After the transition] you will learn life was nothing more than a school; you simply had to pass tests in order to graduate. The one thing everyone has to learn before returning home is unconditional love. If you have learned and practiced this, you have mastered the greatest lesson of all."

~ Elisabeth Kübler-Ross

We all have different life paths, different things that each individual soul has come to learn. While each soul has its own agenda, the one common denominator for each of us is to learn how to love—both ourselves and others (once again, loving ourselves is the hardest part). Seeing the value in everyone, being loving to all things—nature, plants, animals, etc.—and respecting all life are parts of learning to love. What's important is knowing that we are all interconnected, that we are all here together. What one thinks and does affects the others, collectively!

> *I am, because you are. What I do to you, what you do to me, affects the other.*

> *We are all linked together, here on this earth.*

> *It matters what you say and think! It matters to us all! We're all interconnected!*
> ~ Author Unknown

I once heard this very insightful little comment an eight-year-old dying child said to his mother about her anger at God for his terminal illness.

> *God is Love, he is in you and in me; we are one.*

> *If you're mad at God then you're mad at me.*

> *The only thing man can really acquire in this life is an inner awakening. When man opens his heart and strives towards enlightenment, he finds the true meaning*

*of life. The purpose of his existence unfolds.
The only thing that one can leave behind
in life is love for the world. The only thing
that one can bring away is love in one's
heart. They are one and the same.*

~ Master Li—International
Sheng Zhen Society

*Everything was put on this "island," earth,
by the Great Spirit. Created from Love.*

~ Author Unknown

*All people and things are relatives.
Everything is one, the holy men tell us.*

*Although I die, I continue living in
everything that is . . .*

*. . . each thing is everything forever, we are
all one.*

~ Lakota Indians

We are here on earth to know, understand, give,
and accept Love. God is Love. We come to know and
understand God. God is within each of us. We come to
remember and realize who we are, who we were created to
be—not who we are in this body, in this society, but who
we are as souls.

God is Love

~ 1 John 4:8

In order to love, we have to forgive completely, ourselves first and then others.

I WAS IN THE PRESENCE OF AN ANGEL

The following story is about an experience that absolutely drove home for me that life is, truly, all about love.

Joanne and I are soul sisters. Our friendship began many years ago at a Bible study, and though we didn't see each other often, we had an incredible soul connection. When she became pregnant with her thirteenth child, she told me about the health issues this new little one would be facing. I found myself not questioning the arrival of this child, but wondering what the point was for all of the suffering that would certainly be involved, not only for the baby, but also for the family.

The months passed, and I overheard criticism from the community about a thirteenth child. Joanne and I talked a lot during the early months of her pregnancy. I knew this was a difficult task that she, her husband, and her family were taking on with joy. I also knew that it wouldn't be easy on their family in any aspect—financially, emotionally, or spiritually—and yet through it all they were committed to protect this precious life that was conceived from love, who would come to be named Baby Sarah Ann.

Joanne, being an "older mom," underwent extensive testing only to hear that this baby would have birth defects and should be aborted. She was so exhausted with all of the negativity, and I asked her, "What are you going to do with all the information they are telling you? Are you going to have an abortion?" Of course I already knew the answer: "No!"

"Well," I continued, "why have the tests at all then? They are only creating stress and worry for you."

However, wanting the best possible chance for the survival of their baby, she continued to gather information and found the best place to deliver their precious child, which happened to be three hours away from their home. The due date drew near, and it was decided that Sarah would be delivered two weeks early by Cesarean. In doing so, they saved her life as the umbilical cord was wrapped around her neck. She was a tiny four-and-a-half pound precious little girl with two cleft palates.

Two weeks after her birth, Joanne called to say that she and the baby were home, and she asked if I could please come to visit. Joanne told me that Sarah had a disease that the doctors could do nothing for. She wouldn't be able to produce her own blood and would eventually die. She possibly had just two weeks to live, so they sent Baby Sarah Ann home to be with her family.

Arrangements were made for me to visit on Wednesday. Joanne insisted that this life was to be celebrated, and as I drove down their street and up their driveway, there were pink posters plastered everywhere that read, "Welcome

Home, Baby Sarah Ann," with big yellow happy face balloons tied to the bushes and trees!

I arrived with the first two roses from my yard. They bloomed the day Sarah was born. For me, they were symbolic of the love between Sarah and Joanne. I was greeted at the door and noticed that Sarah was in the arms of another couple. As soon as I walked into the room, I instantly felt that I was in the presence of an angel—literally—and I remember saying to myself, "Oh, I know exactly what this is all about. It's about *love*. It's all about love!" That was it! It was crystal clear and just that simple! It was about this couple with twelve other children saying *yes* to God's plan for a thirteenth. I had to wonder how many others of us would have had this kind of courage.

I was allowed the honor of holding Sarah. I noticed her cleft palates, and yet she was beautiful. She reminded me of the characters in *The Phantom of the Opera* or *Beauty and the Beast*—I saw past her physical limitations and directly into her soul. She was magnificently brilliant. How could it have been any different? She was created in the likeness and image of God; she had been perfectly formed. Her older sister stayed sitting next to me, and when Sarah's coloring looked a little blue, she gently took her from me and said, "Sometimes she forgets to breathe and so you just tip her sideways and rub her back." She tilted her little sister just a bit and then tenderly handed her back to me. Joanne asked if I would like to watch how they fed her, and I was both humbled and intrigued to watch this incredible act of love. Sarah ate every two hours for twenty minutes around the clock. Joanne pumped her breasts and then they put the breast milk into a syringe. They used a stethoscope on her chest to make sure the milk was going into her stomach. The milk slowly dripped down the tube and she sucked on her pacifier. It was perhaps the most perfect example of love that I have personally witnessed.

Joanne began to explain Sarah's disease. In about two weeks' time, when Joanne's blood would be completely gone from Sarah's body, she would not be able to make any of her own blood, and then she would die. "Oh, I can't believe that," I began my silent protest to God. "This child is so loved and cared for, she doesn't look like she's leaving us anytime soon!"

It was time for Sarah and Joanne to rest, and I said good-bye with a promise of prayers. I sat in my car in awe as the tears involuntarily streamed down my face. I knew I had witnessed something truly holy.

The following Saturday, I called to leave a message of love and prayers, but when Joanne picked up the phone she said, "Oh, Pati, I guess you heard about Sarah?"

"No," I answered, "what?"

"She died the day after you saw her. I'm so happy that you got to see her."

After we hung up, the tears once again began to flow. I just knew there would be a miracle performed on her behalf. Everyone in the community was praying.

Later, I realized, a miracle had in fact been performed

on behalf of Baby Sarah Ann. Many lives had been touched and would forever be changed because of this family's courage to say *yes* to what was sent to them. From the hospital staff to the clergy support, critics' hearts were softened, people returned to prayer, and many pulled together. I know my life has been changed forever because I was in the presence of an angel.

The day of the funeral, I drove out my driveway and noticed on the road to Joanne's house one last pink sign, complete with a now half-deflated happy face yellow balloon, which read, "Welcome Home, Baby Sarah Ann." I knew it was from God—Welcome Home to Heaven—and I once again felt honored to have witnessed first hand the plan of God.

WE'VE COME TO EXPERIENCE JOY AND FUN . . . YES, IT'S TRUE!!

Joy is the highest energy vibration. Yes, it's true. I've read this many times from an array of different sources. When we feel joy, we exude joy. When we are full of happiness and light, it can simply be by our presence that others will feel this joy and happiness as well.

Negative energy attracts more negative energy, and the same is true with positive energy. This energy can be what we think, say, or do. What we send out to the universe is exactly what we're going to get back. Just like a magnet, we're going to attract toward us whatever we put out.

What generally happens if you say something negative to someone? You will probably get a negative response in return. However, saying something positive will generally reap a positive reaction in return. One smile usually attracts another. Do you find that you are more attracted to someone who is crabby or someone full of joy and smiling? Love, joy, fun—that is how we raise the energy of the earth, and it's also what attracts people to God.

In his book *The True Power of Water*, Dr. Masaru Emoto, a Japanese scientist, author, and visionary, took water droplets, exposed them to various words, music, and environments, and froze them for three hours. He then examined the crystal formations under a dark field microscope and took photographs. Literally, the water droplets changed in formation according to the words and energy around the droplets of water. When someone simply *thought* something positive, like love, happiness, trust, or peace, for example, beautiful shapes were formed in the droplets and the water became beautiful water crystals. The same held true when negative thoughts were brought into the mind, like, fear, hate, greed, or depression. The water crystals took on deformed or unpleasant shapes. Words can simply be written on a piece of paper and taped to the glass and the water is affected. That is how powerful everything we think, say, and do is!

Contrary to what I was taught growing up, I have discovered for myself that there is no virtue in sacrifice or poverty. Wayne Dyer said, "You cannot be sick enough to make one other person well or poor enough to make one other person wealthy or even sad enough to make one other person happy." Only you are responsible for you! You alone are responsible for your happiness and well-being.

When I was in school learning intuitive massage, one of our sessions included a personal reading. An Intuitive Reader (someone gifted in *tuning in*) came and *read* for us the support that we had from the other side. For me, the message came from my guardian angels and my recently deceased dad who ended with, "Don't forget to have fun!" This was a total shock to me, as I thought life was about anything *but* having fun. Fun was something you did on the sly. Working twenty-four-seven was what I thought life was about.

At one point in my life, things had taken a dramatic turn for the worse. I was taking daily drives an hour from home to see my husband in a rehab facility as he was recovering from a stroke. As you can imagine, I was frantically trying to juggle two children still living at home, my job, our business, and the feeling that I needed to see him each day. One day while driving home, a total peace came over me when I noticed a bumper sticker on the car in front of me, which read:

DON'T POSTPONE THE JOY!

This is your life right now . . . not someday when you retire; the children will leave home; time will pass!

Enjoy today!

Chapter 4

SEEING FROM ANOTHER VIEWPOINT

*We have to be willing to let go of our old
belief systems—they served us well.*

~ Father Richard Rohr (Catholic Priest)

It's imperative at some point in our lives that we begin to take responsibility for our own personal beliefs. We cannot simply believe things we were *told* to believe; we must take the inward journey and discover what it is that we personally hold as truth. For me, this involved a lot of letting go. I was always the *yes* person: *Just tell me what you want me to do!* Well, living this philosophy wasn't working for me any longer, and I had to discover a new path for myself. I didn't know which way to go, but thanks to the sacrifices of my mother and my sister, I knew which path I *wasn't* going to take. I wasn't going to follow the path of traditional western medicine. That was the help my mother and sister sought, and they are both dead. So I got out my machete and began hacking a new passageway. In the process of clearing away, I had to do some work around the fact that I had believed what I had been told by others: my parents, teachers, religion, and society. If I was to survive, I had no alternative but to examine what beliefs I had that I could let go of because they just weren't working for me any longer. If I was to continue the way I was, I would just feel like a failure.

By way of example, I'll share a little bit about what I worked through while redefining what I believe. I had always done what I was told, especially by my father. I now realized that his beliefs had been passed down to him, just as mine had been to me. My dad was born during the depression. His parents were divorced. His mother had *men* friends (from my dad's perspective) who apparently didn't like him. At a young age, he ran away from home. My dad married as a young adult, had four children, and thought he was providing well for his family when an unexpected divorce came after eighteen years of marriage and bitterness followed. I began to see that my dad's perception of life was tainted with a lot of negative emotions of rejection and abandonment, and feelings of not being good enough. I realized these beliefs had been passed down to me. I had been living my life by the *family code,* a code that had been created for me by my parents, which had been created for them by their parents. Now it was time for me to decide what was true for me, and what I believed.

One of the most valuable tools I've learned in recent years is the ability to see things from different perspectives. I've come to understand that even though we all have a story, they are told from our own perspectives, which is formed by the generation we're a part of, our upbringing, and our beliefs, experiences, and educations.

> *Sometimes we confuse "beliefs" with "facts."*

Recently, I attended a docent training class at a river near my home. A biologist came to share his experience of the river. "If everyone could see the river through the eyes of a biologist, you'd see a whole other world," he announced upon his arrival. Looking at the river from the eyes of someone merely interested in recreation is totally different than viewing it from the eyes of a biologist. A biologist sees the ecosystems, the sub terrarium, the water, the mammals, the reptiles, and the minerals—the list is endless. Looking at the river from a recreational standpoint, your only concerns may be about beaches, the best swimming hole, where to put the trash, and where to find the outdoor facilities.

What is seen by each of us depends on our backgrounds, histories, and experiences. The biologist's experience of the river is completely different than a recreational user.

*Anything you believe with absolute
certainty is rarely true!*

Let me explain.

I had just flown thirteen hours from Sydney to Los Angeles in business class, courtesy of my daughter who was a flight attendant. On the flight, we were provided with a little overnight bag, which included a toothbrush and toothpaste. I got off this massive airplane, the kind that feels like they have twenty seats across, and went directly to my connecting flight home on a teeny tiny commuter plane, one so small your carry-on luggage had to be checked. I found my seat, which happened to be next to a window. A gentleman was sitting in the aisle seat next to mine. He smiled and got up to let me squeeze my way in. We then had a little light conversation. A bit later, I said something to him and he didn't acknowledge me. I instantly read this and thought, "Oh my gosh, what's wrong with me?" I began spinning as I can do from time to time. "I must smell! I've been on the plane for a long time…no, it's got to be my breath!" The flight attendant came around and I asked for some water, reaching across with every attempt not to lift my arms too high. You remember, the stench…from my armpits! I sat quietly sipping my water (hoping it would clean my breath) until we landed. When we got off the plane, the man smiled and said good-bye. I was still being careful not to get too close! Then I noticed that he offered to help the lady in front of us with her bag, and that she was talking to him but he wasn't answering her either. As he turned, I could see that he was wearing a hearing aid. I spent all that time fretting—*what's wrong with me*—and really it was *what was wrong with him!* The point is that I believed my own assessment very strongly, and it wasn't true at all!

I could tell many stories of *things not being what they seem,* or things I thought were one way which proved not to be that way at all. It was simply my projections of my past experiences that I had brought with me from my life.

One more example comes to mind. I had spent the last three months with my friend's mother in Ireland while they were remodeling her house. It was the first day of frost since I had arrived. It looked like a winter wonderland outside. I wanted to go down the hill into town, so I was driving cautiously. I noticed the contractor working on the house was driving up the hill and making a motion, waving his hands up and down outside his window, signaling *slow down!* When I arrived to town, a text message came in from my friend: *Roads are icy in town; better wait to go to town later in the day.* When I returned home and saw the contractor, I said, "Hi snitch," assuming he had called my friend to tell him I was driving too fast. He explained that he had been on the phone with my friend when he had to hang up because the roads were slick! So there you have it! I thought he had called my friend, but he had only told him about the slick roads that *he* was driving on!

You think you know, but you have no idea!

We're all just people with our own points of view. It doesn't mean one way is right and the other is wrong; it simply means we're different and we learn from each other. Trying to see things from other points of view helps us to have compassion and love more.

Author Paula D'Arcy explains the willingness to see things from a different angle in her book *A New Set of Eyes*. She relays the following conversation between her father and herself in his later years. She'd been in a recent car accident in which her husband and small daughter were killed. Everyone had come to see her in the hospital except the person she had wanted most, her father. Many years had passed and she had come to accept life how it was and not as how she wanted it to be. One day her aging father revealed the truth of why he hadn't come to see her. He was so grief-stricken that he couldn't find the hospital. He had driven for hours, asking for directions, but eventually he could only find his own house. Paula D'Arcy shares, "I was left looking directly at the judgments I had held so righteously: realizing that what I had believed to be true was not at all what was and yet I had believed it so intensely."

Change the way you look at things and the things you look at will change

~ Wayne Dyer

Wisdom comes from pathways you've walked in another person's moccasins.

~ Author Unknown

Misperceptions produce fear.
True perceptions foster love.

~ Author Unknown

WORDS ARE JUST WORDS: DIFFERENT WORDS ~ SAME MEANING ~ NEW PERSPECTIVE

For a moment, let's think of all the words that people use to refer to the process of the soul leaving the body: death, dying, going to heaven, passed on, passed on to the next world, crossed over, after life, next life, the other side, finished your earth walk. I'm sure you can think of many others. My personal favorite, however, is *transitioning.*

Running through this litany of words we have for *dying,* I remembered a retreat that I had attended where a priest shared with me a story about a woman in *transition* in the emergency room.

He recalled, "I was summoned to the emergency room to give the last rites to someone about to die. I walked up and down the hall looking for the person I was to see. I noticed a woman in one room lying naked on a gurney. At first glance it looked to me like she was about to give birth, but upon closer observation, I could see that she was, in fact, about to give birth, but not to a baby. She was birthing into the after life!" This was a real revelation for this priest. This statement was also very intriguing to me. Birthing into this life and birthing out of this life can look the same! The soul leaving the body is a birthing process; birth and death are two words describing the same transition in the circle of life.

> *Death is not the opposite of life. Life has no opposite.*
> *The opposite of death is birth. Life is eternal.*
>
> ~ Eckert Tolle

After my mother died, I spoke about her death to a Native American healer. She stopped me in midsentence, looked me directly in the eye, and said, "Your mother didn't die, she simply *crossed over*," and I knew deep down that this was a *truth* that I believed! I had seen my mother's leaving this earth as *dying*, and the healer had seen it simply as *transitioning to the other side*. Once again, different words describing the same phenomenon.

Here is one more example of how the use of different words, or seeing things from another person's viewpoint, can have a positive and peaceful effect.

While on an extended trip to Ireland, I was staying with my friend's eighty-year-old mother, Martha. She anxiously awaited the daily news on the radio because the recent deaths were announced. It always began, "Radio Clare has been informed of the following deaths." Each time I would add, "What they should say is, 'Radio Clare has been informed of the following rebirths!'" Martha often commented that she wondered who would be listening to the announcement upon her death. Martha is a trendsetter from way back, and so we wrote an announcement for the radio to announce her *rebirth* when the time came.

> *"Hello. It's me, Martha. Being the visionary and trendsetter that I am, wish to share with the community of Clare my joy. Last night, my soul was called home to be with God and loved ones who have gone before me, to heaven. It was an incredibly beautiful and peace-filled experience, brilliant! Please join my precious children and grandchildren, who are my delight, in the celebration of my life and the journey of my soul into the next life for all eternity, by attending my Requiem Mass to be held on _____ at, _____ celebrated by my son. I end with this: An Irish saying that we put on the family headstone many years ago!"*

> *Ni crioch ach athfhas ~ It's not the end . . . it's a new beginning!*

When we had finished composing the announcement, an old song came to mind, and I sang the chorus to Martha: "Closing time; every new beginning comes from some other beginning's end!"

EXPERIENCING SPIRITUAL SUPPORT FROM ANOTHER POINT OF VIEW
(Learning to Read the Signs)

If there *is* life after death, then it would make sense that we would be able to communicate with the ones who have made the transition to the next life, if we simply knew how to *tune in*. It is much like turning the dial on the radio to find the right frequency, getting rid of all the static and noise. I think it is like being in school. Classroom learning comes easily for some, but for others it takes more effort. It is the same with learning to *tune in*. Some people have a gift, while others have to work harder at developing it. Some people *see*, others *hear*, others *know*. The point is that everyone can develop sensitivity to the help and support provided from all heaven and earth, including nature, the ones who have gone before us, our spiritual helpers (or guardian angels), Saints, and Ascended Masters (the holy men and women who are already in heaven, including Jesus and Mary).

We can pay attention to the help and support from the ones on the other side (heaven) simply by being still, quieting our minds, and listening. This is very different than *praying*. Sometimes in prayer we have a tendency to tell God how we think he should do his job! We're in *action mode*. But listening requires a *stillness* of the mind. Sometimes it's not even so much about being physically still, it's just about mentally clearing the head.

I find that I can't easily be physically still. I *listen* much better when I'm walking or doing some kind of mundane chore or driving long distances alone. These are the things that tend to free my mind.

Signs are another way I am aware of the support from the other side. What do I mean by *signs*? I pay attention to the words or songs that come on the radio or the television. I look at billboards; I watch the clouds, study the trees, and pay attention to what animals cross my path. When anything comes to my awareness, I ask myself, *Is this support from the other side?*

Here are a couple of examples to help you catch a glimpse of what *reading the signs* can look like:

I feel Divine Support in everyday things like wind chimes gently blowing in the wind (to me these are angels) or a when a gust of wind blows through the treetops (to me these are spirits).

On a visit to Washington to see my daughter, we were having a bout of bad weather. I had been at her place for about a week and I was ready for my drive home to California. But all the weather reports had advised against it, as another round of storms were due to come in. I knew that I would be away from my home for at least another week if I stayed. I had been practicing *tuning in,* so I began by *checking in with myself.* (How am I feeling? Is my body tense or relaxed?) Finally, I felt a sense of calm, the *yes* emerged, and I made the decision to leave. All went well until I reached the pass to cross the mountains from Oregon to California. It began to snow ever-so lightly, but I knew that meant heavier snow over the summit. I stopped for gas. Why? I really didn't need any. (I was later to discover that it was all about the *timing.*) I asked the store clerk about the conditions for crossing the summit and then began the journey upward. As I began the climb, it started to snow harder. I had chains with me, but I couldn't imagine having to do anything more unpleasant than putting them on the car! It was cold out there! Drivers were beginning to pull off the road to chain up, and just as I thought I might have to give in and do the same, a snowplow made a u-turn right in front of me! I followed the snowplow up the summit and down the other side. The song on the radio caught my attention, "I Just Called to Say I Love You." I knew it was support from the other side. How did I know? It brought tears to my eyes and I trusted that I just *knew.*

It took me a while before I was able to accept and see my spiritual support from another point of view. I began to become open to the fact that God and the angels can connect with us in myriad ways. By my willingness to see things differently than what I had been familiar with, and by waiting and watching for the *signs*, I had a clear, safe passage home.

Chapter 5

DYING AND THE AFTERLIFE: A DIFFERENT PERSPECTIVE

We are Spirits with a body for this little blurp in time we call life!

In his book *The Power Of Intention,* Wayne Dyer speaks of two possible scenarios for how a person could feel about death. The first says that we're physical bodies that are born and we go on to live for a while; then ultimately we deteriorate, our flesh wears out, then we die and are dead forever. Or, as my Irish friend Martha put it, "When you're dead you're dead and that's that!"

The second point of view says, very simply, that we're eternal, an infinite soul in a temporary expression of flesh. Another way to say it is: We're souls for eternity, here in physical bodies for this little bit of time we call *life.*

Death is simply a shedding of the physical body, like a snake sheds its skin, like butterflies shed their cocoons, or like hermit crabs leave their shells behind. Death is a transition to a higher state of awareness. Death is not an aspect of life; life continues on without end. We are just here in bodies for this little blurp in time that we call life. The dying of the body is just a *part* of the journey of the soul.

In his book *Still Here,* Ram Dass answers the question, "Will we personally exist this way after death?" He explains, "If we subscribe to a materialistic view of things and believe ourselves to be nothing more than our body and ego, the answer is almost certainly no, Richard Alpert, a.k.a. Ram Dass, will cease to be when this body has stopped breathing. But if we have expanded our consciousness to include the Soul and awareness levels, we understand that the physical organism is merely the shell, the rented apartment. Knowing myself to be a Soul, I realize that something will indeed survive death, though this body and personality will be gone." (Added note: I personally believe the personality won't be gone.)

Ram Dass continues, "In India, life is seen as a single part in a book, not the entire tome; death is viewed as a transformative experience, not the end."

> *If eternal life can be lost . . . it can't be eternal!*

Christians believe in eternity, or at least we say we do, but we never talk about it. In fact, "*When you're dead you're dead and that's that!"* is a kind of philosophy among many Christians. My experience has been that while many may say they believe in eternity, they actually don't believe that they are really going to heaven because of all the things they perceive that they did wrong in their life, or because of the things they didn't do well enough! I find that it's not talked about a lot of the time because there is no feeling of hope for seeing heaven or God. The thought may be, 'If we don't talk about it, it will just go away!'

> *Eternity is not the hereafter; this is it.*
>
> ~ Joseph Campbell

This is eternity. We are living it; we're part of it. Eternity is right now; it has no beginning and no end. The dictionary defines the word eternity as timeless; infinite time; duration without beginning or end. **Infinite means a timeless existence**.

> *We are not human beings having a spiritual experience.*
> *We are spiritual beings having a human experience.*
>
> ~ Pierre Teilhard de Chardin

DEATH DOES NOT END LIFE... HOW DO YOU KNOW? DID YOU DO IT? DIE, I MEAN...

People often comment to me that when we're alive, we don't know anything about dying because we haven't done it yet. But that's not actually true. There are many stories and books of people who have had *near-death* experiences and have lived to tell about them. So we do know that there is life after death. There are stories like the ones I'm about to share with you from everyday people. Then there are people like Elisabeth Kübler-Ross, who have done scientific research on dying and life after death. All we have to do is to soften our hearts, let go of our preconceived notions, and be open to other possibilities.

Georgia's Story
Age 76, practicing Catholic

Georgia and I have been friends for many years. She and her husband, Dick, were with my dad during his illness. We talked a lot about death and dying at that time, and she told me the story of her near-death experience on more than one occasion. During the writing of this book, I called her to hear it once again, and this is how it goes:

> I was pregnant with Larry, my second son. Dick was at work and I laid down on the couch to try to sleep as I had a terrible pain in the back of my

neck, an excruciating pain. I pleaded with God to please take the pain away, but it didn't go away, and so I pleaded with Him, "If you can't take the pain away then take me away!"

Soon after that, I felt myself floating above my body and I could see my body lying on the couch. Then I saw a tunnel. There were beautiful clouds and rays of light streaming toward me. Then I saw Jesus walking through the tunnel toward me.

"Have I died?" I asked Him. "If you want to," He answered. "Will the pain continue if I return?" "Yes," he answered. "Well then let's go," I replied, as I motioned toward the tunnel. Just then I heard my first-born son, Michael, cry. I looked at Jesus with a heavy heart and said, "I can't leave him!" Tears began to well in my eyes and my voice began to crack. "I can't leave him!" I said again. With that, I floated back down to my body and attended to Michael.

"Was the pain gone?" I asked. "Yes," she answered. Then she continued, "I have never been afraid to die from that moment on. There is life after death, I saw it first hand!

Here are a couple of stories other people have shared with me about their personal experiences:

Jane and her husband went to visit their grandson in the hospital. He was dying, but before he left his body permanently, he went to the Light and returned before his final departure. She asked who was there, and he said, "We all are." Jane told me this story with tears in her eyes.

Debra was sailing when her boat capsized. She said that she saw *the tunnel*. It was iridescent, pearl white, bright, smooth, and shiny. She repeated the words *light, pearly, and iridescent* several times. The tunnel was on her left side and on her right side she saw the boat house where her three-year-old daughter was. She made a conscious decision to stay, but added that she wasn't afraid to die.

You too will hear these stories if you are open to the conversation. I didn't solicit these accounts; they were freely told to me.

> *Do you see, oh my brothers and sisters, it is not chaos and death.*
>
> *It is form and union and plan. It is eternal life. It is happiness.*
>
> ~ Emerson

ANOTHER WAY TO SEE DEATH ~ WE'RE SIMPLY TRANSFORMED

Learn to appreciate the beauty in all parts of life's journey!

I was taking a walk when a large pile of plant prunings caught my attention. I noticed that it was just lying there, apparently waiting. *Waiting for what?* I wondered. Waiting to be transformed! These plant clippings were just resting, waiting for the continuation of their journey, to become transformed into compost. Though it will be the same material, it will have a different look. So it is with our spirits; they will be the same even after dying changes the body. However, the spirit will continue to live.

While driving in Ireland with Martha one day, we passed a clump of trees when she said, "What's wrong with those trees? They all look dead." That statement caught my attention, as it was just beginning to turn to fall and certainly the trees were beginning to lose their leaves. But I also knew that while they appeared to be dying, (as is the illusion of death), the sap in the trees and the roots was very much alive (as is the soul), just waiting, resting, storing energy, preparing for spring when a rebirthing would take place.

This is the same process acorns go through, dropping off the trees and falling to the ground to wait through the winter quietly, lingering, resting, and waiting for spring when they become a new little sprout. The oak tree and the sprout are the same, just in different forms. It's true for a butterfly as well. It begins as a caterpillar and then spins itself into a cocoon, waiting until it is released as a beautiful butterfly. It is the circle of life, which we are all a part of.

> *Exactly as in dying, the body has been shed; the soul is free to fly.*

While house-sitting for a friend, I watched *The Lion King*. Mufasa, the king, explains to his young son, Simba, about the circle of life. "We lions eat the antelope, the antelope eat the grass, and when our bodies die, they become fertilizer for the grass to grow; its just part of the circle of life."

GONE FROM MY SIGHT

> *I am standing upon the seashore. A ship at my side spreads her white sails to the morning breeze and starts for the blue ocean.*
>
> *She is an object of beauty and strength. I stand and watch her until at length she hangs like a speck of white cloud just*

where the sea and sky come to mingle with
each other.

Then someone at my side says: "There . . .
she is gone!"

"Gone where?"

Gone from my sight, that is all. She is just
as large in mast and hull and spar as she
was when she left my side and she is just as
able to bear her load of living freight to her
destined port.

Her diminished size is in me, not in her,
and just at the moment when someone at
my side says: "There, she is gone!" There
are other eyes watching her coming, and
other voices watching her coming, and
other voices ready to take up the glad
shout: "Here she comes!"

And that is dying.

~ Henry Van Dyke

*You've been fearful of being absorbed in
the ground or drawn up by the air.*

*Now, your water bead lets go and drops
into the ocean, where it came from.*

*It no longer has the form it had, but it is
still water.*

*The essence is the same. This giving up is
not a repenting.*

It's a deep honoring of yourself.

~ Rumi

The Birth that is Death – Life after Life
~ Father Joe Kempf,
No One Cries the Wrong Way

Once there were twins in their mother's womb. They were
very happy there, for it was warm and cozy and safe. They
played games all day and often stayed up late into the night
telling stories. Sometimes they were quiet, simply listening
to each other's heartbeats and enjoying the comfort of each
other's presence.

One day, there was tremendous upheaval and great

turmoil. When things settled down a bit and the one twin opened his eyes again, he saw to his horror that his brother was gone. He was both frightened and heartbroken. Not only was this his twin that was gone but also his best friend. Now he was alone. Now, he no longer had his brother with whom to play games. He had no one with whom to stay up late into the night and tell stories. How empty the womb seemed now, how dark and lonely.

What he did not realize was that his brother had been born! He could not see the loving arms that were there to welcome his brother at his birth. He did not see the tears of joy in his mother and father's eyes that their child had been born to them. He did not really understand what it meant to "be born." All he knew was that his brother was gone and the world seemed terribly empty and sad.

So it is for us with the death of a loved one. When someone we love dies, our world seems empty and cold. We think our loved one should be there.

> *Death is nothing more than a migration of*
> *the soul from this place to another.*
>
> ~ Plato

WE'RE ALL GOING TO HEAVEN!
IS THIS DIFFERENT THAN YOU THOUGHT?

We know because God told us.

~ John 14:1-6

Jesus said to His disciples:

Do not let your hearts be troubled. Have faith in God and faith in me. In My Father's house there are many dwelling places; otherwise, how could I have told you that I was going to prepare a place for you?

> *I am indeed going to prepare a place for you, and then I shall come back to take you with Me, that where I am you also may be.*

Feeling like we're all going to heaven may be a difficult concept to comprehend for some of us. I grew up not feeling worthy of ever reaching heaven. When I was a young convert to the Catholic religion, a young (and I thought a bit arrogant) priest told me, "I'm going to heaven! It's a decision I've made!" I didn't understand what he was talking about at the time. However, since then, I've begun to see that I am loved simply because I am, and I cannot earn my way to heaven, and I too am going to heaven.

God is not trying to keep us from Him. We are created in the likeness and image of God. God created us to be with Him. He doesn't get out his scorecard and continually make checks for all the things we do wrong—things *we perceive* we do wrong. There is nothing we can do to earn God's love and there is nothing we can do to have God's love taken away. It is simply a gift. When you think about a *loving* family, do the mother and father embrace their children or push them away? No matter what our kids do, speaking from personal experience as a parent, we always welcome them to be with us.

You may remember the story of the Prodigal Son. It's a parable that Jesus told of a man who has two sons. The younger son wants his family inheritance early. He then sets off to a far away land and squanders the money on wild living. When the money runs out, he has to take a job feeding pigs. Finally, he has the courage to go home and ask for his father's forgiveness. The father has been waiting, and welcomes his son back with open arms, overjoyed that his son has returned.

Was the son kept from his father? Absolutely not. His father was overjoyed at his return! And God has an even greater love for us, a love that is far grander than human love. His love is *Agape,* unconditional love. Love without condition. That's all that needs to be said!

Don't waste your precious time trying to figure out the murderers, people who are bad (according to the perception of you or society). Let God be God and relax in the fact that you don't have to know. All we're concerned with here is *you* and *you are going to heaven.* It is your birthright; it is a grace.

> " . . . *yet standing before Christ I marveled that he did not judge me at all. He knew the tiniest remote thing about me and accepted me just as I was. He even delighted in me!*"
>
> ~ Betty Eadie, *Embraced by the Light*

A LETTER I WROTE TO MY DAD FROM GOD WHEN I FOUND OUT THAT HE WAS DYING

I had been to a workshop with author Terry Hershey and I adapted the concept I heard there about a new, gentler look at a merciful and loving God. I wanted to give my dad a sense of what I had received from Terry's perspective of a more compassionate God—much different than we had been taught.

> Hi Sam,
> It's me, you know, "The Man Upstairs!" The news you just received from the doctor—that you have renal failure—sounds scary, huh? Would you believe it if I told you, Sammy my boy, that actually it's my gift to you and your family! When you think about all the possible ways to leave this

earth, renal failure is very gentle. Cancer has also been called a gift from Me: a gift of time—time to get things in order, time to say good-bye (where I'll see you on the other side ☺). But with kidney failure, there isn't the pain. No Sam, you've learned suffering and giving; well, now it's time for the completion of the circle: joy and receiving.

The lesson on this final part of the journey home is about letting go. I promise I'll catch you! It's about giving others the opportunity to be there for you, like you've always been there for them. You need not worry about anything, that's what they pay me for! ☺. I know of your desires to be self-sufficient—that's another reason for the diagnosis. You can be self-sufficient, but do you want to be alone? Maybe you do, and you get to pick. Nobody knows when anyone's time on earth is up, and so a favorite saying comes to mind: "Even if I knew the world would end tomorrow, I'd still plant my cherry tree today!" Don't give up. Do what you feel like doing: sleep, rest, go to town, whatever you want to do. Contrary to what some believe, life is about joy. *Don't postpone the joy!*

And one more thing, Sam my man, I assure you that I am not the God you fear. I have no score card. I love you simply because I do. You were made in the likeness and image of Me—how could it be different? The things you did that you felt didn't quite measure up, they weren't a problem for Me. I didn't even notice. Life on earth is about learning; failure is simply the opportunity to begin again, more intelligently, the next time. All the good things you did, well, once again, I didn't notice. I have no score card. I just enjoyed them. There is nothing you can do to earn My love, there's nothing you can do to make Me not love you—it's simply a grace.

Sammy, I promise you a peaceful crossing over. You've made it easy by not wanting to be hooked up to machines. All you have to do when you're ready is to simply let go. I'll catch you; I've not left you yet. It's puzzling to me why everyone resists coming home. Just think of family Christmases. Remember the anticipation you felt while waiting for those you love who were coming home to celebrate. Well, that's it exactly! I'm simply looking forward to your returning home and into my arms.

We'll have the biggest party ever! You'll come and sit by Me on My big white throne and we'll have us a good practice laugh (what you do best ☺) before we really get this party started! The angels and ancestors will be here cheering. We've been waiting for you! And I'll smile and say, "This is my son Sam with whom I'm pleased!

Part 2

Being Present
With Those in
Transition

Chapter 6

TIPS FOR FRIENDS, CAREGIVERS, AND ADULT CHILDREN

If you find yourself in the situation of taking care of someone who is getting on in years, or perhaps your loved one has gotten the news that their days are limited, it can be as much of a shock to you as it is to them. Sometimes the timeline for transitioning can take years, and other times it's very short. For me, it was nineteen days from the day that my mother was diagnosed with throat cancer until the day she died. My dad, on the other hand, was diagnosed with renal failure, and we had six months before he transitioned out.

In both cases, it was a relatively short time to put my life *on hold* to be with my parents. When my mother was diagnosed, I still had two boys at home in high school. My two girls were in college, and I was working full-time at the church, was married, and was a business owner. However, with my dad, my children were grown and out of the house. I was no longer married and was on disability because of surgery, so my time was a bit easier to juggle. Through all of this, I learned that not everyone is supposed to be a caregiver. We all have our gifts that we offer to the world. The following are lessons that I learned while I was with my parents and others during the end of their lives. Whether you are an adult child of a dying parent, a caregiver, or both, there may be some tips here that will work for you.

OUR RESPONSIBILITY FOR TAKING CARE OF OTHERS

I'm sad to say that when my mother wanted to move up north to be close to me, I was less than thrilled about the prospect. I remember thinking, *I took care of you your whole life—when do you get to take care of yourself?* I asked a nun at church, "Just what is my responsibility for my mother?" Much to my surprise and delight she answered, "It's not your responsibility to take care of your mother. It is simply your responsibility to be sure that she is taken care of."

Sometimes we can't do for our family members what we wish we could. Trust that you are doing exactly what you are supposed to be doing. Family members often don't share their life experiences with those that are close, or with those they love. Perhaps they can, however, speak freely with someone other than kin. This has proven true for me on more than one occasion. Oftentimes, family members feel they have an image to uphold, so they don't feel free to be totally honest. What I'm trying to say is that you may be the caregiver of a loved one, but if you're not, don't feel guilty. Not everyone is called to be a caregiver.

> *It is simply your responsibility to be sure that they are taken care of.*

NOT EVERYONE IS CALLED TO BE A CAREGIVER

The story of Christopher Reeves, the movie star who played Superman, comes to mind. After his tragic accident that left him a quadriplegic, his wife stated that she did not do any of the daily care for Christopher; she was his wife, not his nurse. I thought this statement was a significant thing to say, and that she served as a role model to the rest of us. Just because someone you love is ill doesn't mean you need to give up your life. As a matter of fact, you shouldn't give up your life. When you are fresh, you are better able to cope. What's best for you is best for those around you!

Remember, not everyone is *called* to be the caregiver of a parent or loved one. It doesn't mean you're *good* if you had the opportunity to take care of another and doesn't mean you're *bad* if you didn't. I believe that sometimes, unexplained things are simply soul contracts that come from a Higher Source.

What's best for you is best for those around you!

KEEP EVERYTHING POSITIVE

When your loved one says anything that is negative, turn it into a positive, especially when they say negative things about themselves. Help them to get rid of the voices in their heads that say, "You're not trying hard enough, you're not doing enough, you're not good enough." I know this works, even though it takes a while to change the bad habit.

While I was staying with my friend Martha, it was six weeks before I heard her begin to say positive things about the weather, or before she would give herself permission to rest. It's important for the one who's dying to see another viewpoint. It's important to give our own opinions instead of agreeing with what they say just to keep the peace. The final transition is a very important time of learning for the one who's dying; maybe they will get lessons they weren't able to get in earlier years.

I experienced this firsthand with my dad. It was just days before he left his body when I had the courage to say to him, "Dad, I'm not sure if you know this, but you don't treat me very nice." He was horrified. For seventy-seven years, he had no idea! No one, including me, ever had the nerve to tell him. He truly felt terrible! He simply treated me and other women the way he had seen women being treated in his youth. I continued by saying, "It's not just your issue, Dad, it's mine as well. I never stood up for myself." The next morning I found a note he had tried to write on the dining room table with his Mason Ring lying on top of it. The only thing I could read on it was, "Good Pati." I went to his room and asked him what the note said and what was up with his ring. He said the note was to thank everyone for their love and kindness and the ring was for my son.

When they say anything that is negative,
help them turn it into something positive!

BE SILLY, HAVE FUN ~ NO IMAGES TO MAINTAIN

Try to do things that are fun! Even when they resist, keep plugging away. My friend Martha and I had the best time when we were together. She let loose, and we sang and were silly. I wasn't family, so she had no image to maintain. She would roll her eyes at me, and we would laugh together. Martha used a walker, and when she got up in the mornings I could hear her begin to stir from down the hall. That was my cue to open the kitchen door and call to her from the kitchen, "Martha O'Leary . . . Come on down!" as if she were a contestant on The Price is Right. She would laugh so hard that she couldn't take another step. I sang and danced around her, massaged her head and face, and kissed her forehead. It was fun to see her lighten up as the time passed. It was then that I recognized the fact that older people are just children in reverse.

My daughter recently emailed me about a massage class she had observed. She said she felt *called* to maternal and elder massage. It was verification for me that I had been right. What the elders need is the same as what a baby needs. I noticed that older people need the nurturing they maybe didn't receive as children, especially coming from large families. Affection was not something that was given freely in my family. I know that Martha loved to be touched and that a head and face massage was non-threatening, loving, and nurturing. Hugging, well now that's another story! (In my experience, I've found that sometimes hugging feels too close for many, where gentle massage can more easily be received.)

Elderly people are just children in reverse!

SAY WHAT YOU NEED TO SAY

Saying what you need to say is healing not only for the two of you in the present, but also for the lineage on both ends: past and future. The soul work that you do benefits seven generations, forward and back!

My mother and I had some intimate talks in the middle of the night at the hospital toward the end. I would go very early in the morning when her medication was due. I found out things about her that she had trouble acknowledging in her life. We talked about things we had not talked about or said before, things that were painful for us both, yet very therapeutic. Those days were very intense, but they were also a real opportunity for growth and healing for both of us.

Take advantage of clear, direct communication!

DON'T TAKE ANYTHING PERSONALLY ~ PUT ON YOUR FILTER!

Taking care of a family member is hard; you may not be *seen,* or perhaps even appreciated. They know the buttons to push and you have history together. Don't take it personally. Put on your filter and just keep plugging away. I was with my friend's auntie during her last months, and when I left, she called to tell her daughter *how holy I was.* Certainly it wasn't true; it was just the illusion of my being holy. I was no different than her niece, I just wasn't family.

A prophet is never appreciated at home.

DON'T TAKE THE ANGER OF ANOTHER PERSONALLY

This is particularly important with relatives or siblings who are also impacted by the death of your mutual loved one. They may be angry at the downturn of the health of a parent or family member. Remember, it's only fear that brings us to this point. The fear of losing our loved one may cause us to look for someone to blame. Their anger with you is just displaced from themselves. There can be a sense of helplessness.

My mother was dying of throat cancer, and I had been the one to call my brother in Missouri to tell him he should come to see her if he wanted to see her while she was still living. He and his wife made the long drive from

Missouri to California. When they arrived, they began to tell me that I wasn't doing enough (acting through fear) and that I was tired of taking care of her. Their perception was that I wanted her to die. Well, needless to say, my feelings were hurt, but I was brave enough to say, "The reality is that Mom is dying and the goal now is to keep her comfortable." I then left, leaving them the space to cope with their feelings.

As I work with the families of people in transition, I find time and again that the adult children have the hardest time. While visiting George, it was his caregiver son who was distressed when I talked frankly with George about his transition. On a surface level he knew George wanted to die, but there it was, right out in the open, and I was talking about it! There is generally someone in every family who is unable to acknowledge the changes that are happening. When things begin to shift, it affects everyone. So anger at the thought of losing a loved one is quite normal. Their life too will change, and change can be scary.

Remember: It's not about you personally. Certainly there will be a chance for family issues to be resolved, and you will just become a mirror for those family members to see themselves more clearly. You are just a facilitator for the transition, holding sacred space.

> *Put on your filter ~ It's not about you personally!*

TAKE CARE OF YOURSELF, GUILT FREE!

It is extremely important that you take care of yourself. Sometimes I just excuse myself and go to my room and read, write, sleep, talk to a friend, and now and then have a good cry. It's very therapeutic! A drive by myself is always healing for me, too. I then feel fresh and ready to begin once again.

Don't take abuse from the one dying or from the ones visiting them. Abuse comes in many forms. It may be as simple as something not *feeling very nice*. If someone seems irritated or upset, ask them about it directly; it will defuse the situation. While it is important to let them have their space, don't try to fix it or make it better for them. Don't read into it. It's not personal. Don't forget the adjustment that they are also having to deal with. Their earthly life is coming to an end, or their parent or sibling is leaving them.

> *Just go and take care of yourself—do something fun, guilt free!*

KEEP YOUR BOUNDARIES STRONG AND CLEAR

Remember, you're not a doormat! If you're a family member, buttons will get pushed. I believe it's part of the soul contract. Pushing buttons is a way of the dying one's saying, "I'm getting ready to leave this earth. I'm giving you another opportunity to stand up for yourself, to stand strong! Will you take it?" Maybe this lesson is for you or it could be for someone else. By your standing up for yourself, you are role-modeling for others. Don't cave in! Don't *gut through* a situation, thinking *it's nearly over, I can put up with this abuse* (however slight) *until they're gone.* Trust me, the issues will remain until you resolve them, even after the loved one is gone. Give others an opportunity to grow and find your personal power by standing up for yourself. (Not in anger but from a place of gratitude and love.)

My dad wanted me to stay with him in his house for his final days, and I really struggled, asking myself, *Why Pati? Why can't you stay with him?* On my way to town an armadillo sauntered across the street. In the Native American spiritual tradition, the armadillo represents boundaries. I understood that this was a message for me to *keep my boundaries strong and clear.* When I returned to my father's house, I was very clear that I couldn't stay. "Dad, I have to leave tomorrow. You are welcome to come with me, or I'll be back in a few days, but I have to go for now. Take the rest of the day to think about what you would like to do, and you can let me know tomorrow." (Man, was that ever hard!) What's best for you is best for those around you. (By the way, he decided to come with me! An opportunity for growth for both of us.)

Do only what you can do with joy!

DON'T PUSH YOUR AGENDA

Resist the temptation that you know what is best for the person going through transition—what they need to read, hear, or do. Trust they will get the information and knowledge they need. Sometimes it happens when you least expect it, even when they're asleep.

While I was in a class in Hawaii, (a very laid-back learning environment), there was one exhausted young mother who clearly needed rest. She had her eyes closed for much of the teachings. Much to her surprise, on the last day, she along with everyone else was able to talk about the lessons of the week. She had received exactly what she needed simply by being present. We just need to trust that others and ourselves are receiving whatever it is that our souls need, even when we don't think things are happening according to our expectations. When I worked in ministry, I was fond of saying: "I did the preparation, but it's not my party, its God's party, and I just have to rest in the fact that He's in control. Those who are supposed to be there will be. Whatever anyone gets from it, they will get." How easy is that!

Resist the temptation that you know what is best for others!

REMAIN A PART OF THE *TRIBE*

Talk their language. This isn't a time to try and convert anyone. It's not your business. I'm not suggesting that you avoid meaningful conversations, but arguing over theories or language doesn't seem prudent. While in Ireland, I saw many grottos and holy wells, at least one in every town, in fact. They really weren't speaking to me until my priest friend told me they were *Healing Energy Places*. Well now! That was a language I could relate to. They were the same places where prayer is offered and answered, no matter what words were used. He used language I could understand and that was meaningful to me, which drew me in. If he would have insisted on a narrow use of verbiage, I wouldn't have been open to experiencing these very holy sites.

> *Be open and flexible with the words*
> *another uses.*

ENCOURAGE ~ DON'T PUSH

Offer encouragement, but don't push. Because of our own fear and our not wanting to deal with the reality of losing our loved one, we may simply think they're not trying hard enough.

Remove any obstacles that can be used as an excuse. For instance, "I would walk more, but it's raining." You may suggest taking a walk inside, or even simply standing up several times.

Explain the benefits: "If you want your body to continue to work, you'll have to use it." A consequence they may not have considered is that social services may intervene if they think you're not capable or being well taken care of.

Be sure they understand the consequences: "I'm happy to walk with you, but I am not happy to push you in a wheel chair because you don't want to exercise. I will do what you need to have done, but I will not do things that you can do for yourself! If I do, I will just feel used."

However, when all is said and done, respect their decision. Trust the inner knowing of their body, their life's journey. Honor what their body wants and needs. Trust that their body knows exactly what to do. If they feel tired, let them rest. If they feel like sleeping, let them do that. If they want to stop eating, honor that. Give them permission to listen to their instincts instead of what you say or society says. Certainly there is balance here. Remember the saying, *You can lead a horse to water, but you can't make it drink!*

The main thing here is that how they decide to live their life shouldn't affect how you live yours.

It was close to Christmas when I was staying with Martha. I brought in a small holly tree in a pot from outside. I told her I thought we should decorate it for a bit of Christmas spirit. She made it clear that she was having nothing to do with it. I said, "Okay, but I'm going to decorate for Christmas." She loved being the director. I didn't push her. I simply stated what it was that I was going to do.

> *Remove any obstacles that can be used as an excuse.*

FIND COMPASSION

Remember, death is just another *transition* in life. The person going through the transition is preparing for a trip. It's the journey of their soul, and they need extra rest and the permission of loved ones to do so. They are storing energy for the journey back to God, a simple rebirthing of the soul. Just think of what a baby needs—touching, caring, rest, food. That is what a person *birthing* into the next life needs as well.

> *Have compassion and respect for their wishes.*

> *Trust they know what is best for them.*

DON'T RUN THE LIFE OF ANOTHER

Don't think you know what's best for another—you don't. Don't act out of good intentions. Ask first, and include them as much as possible. *Do not* take over *their* life. Don't run interference for God, trying to protect them from pain. (This most often manifests when caregivers choose to not tell them the truth of a situation.)

When I was working for the church, I finally hired myself an assistant. She was very efficient and began doing many things I hadn't asked her to do, and I began to feel pushed out. When I was asked in spiritual direction, "What would have made that better for you?" I knew instantly, "To have been asked!"

Do not take over their *life!*

ASK THEM IF THERE IS ANYTHING THEY STILL WANT TO DO

This simple offering is an important element not to be overlooked. Sometimes, before the one in transition feels complete, there may be projects that they feel are incomplete. Simply by asking, "Are there any things that you feel are unfinished or any places or people you would still like to see?"

One client had an unfinished quilt that she had been working on, and she had regrets that she wasn't going to complete it. When asked if she had anyone who could help finish her project, she gave us names of friends who may be willing to lend a hand. Being reassured that others were willing to help gave her a true sense of peace, knowing that her heirloom would be completed. It also gave her friends an opportunity to share in her dream.

My ninety-year-old friend wanted to visit her birth home in Missouri. I removed all of the obstacles for her by volunteering to accompany her on her trip. She was able to see where she had grown up and returned to her home in California with a new sense of contentment and serenity.

GIVE THEM PERMISSION TO LEAVE

Assure them that everyone and everything will be taken care of when they're gone. Reassure them of their legacy. Don't joke with them, trying to ease the situation with statements like, "You can't die now, I don't have time to bury you!" What they need is support to leave this earth when the time comes. Talk about your feelings of missing them after they're gone, but be sure they know you and everyone and everything they leave behind will be fine.

Tell them in a non-joking manner that it is safe for them to leave whenever they choose.

LET'S REVIEW

⭐ **See that your loved one is taken care of:** Not everyone is *called* to be a caregiver.

⭐ **Keep everything positive:** For everyone including yourself.

Have fun, be silly ~ no images to maintain: Have fun, sing and dance, laugh then laugh some more!

Say what you need to say: Don't hold back things that need to be said; they're healing for everyone!

Don't take anything personally: Put on your filter.

Don't take the anger of another personally: Give others the space to deal with their own issues!

Take care of yourself…guilt free: Be sure to make time to rejuvenate yourself!

Keep your boundaries clear: Do only what you can do with a happy heart!

Don't feel guilty: You owe your life to no one!

Don't push your agenda: Trust that others know what is best for them!

Remain a part of the *tribe*: Don't try to get others to see things your way! Speak their language.

Encourage—don't push: Make suggestions, be available, but don't push.

⭐ **Find Compassion:** Remember they are simply preparing for a journey back to God.

⭐ **Be clear in your communications—crystal clear:** Leave no room for doubt. Ask questions.

⭐ **Don't run the life of another:** Trust that you don't have to do it all to keep the world from falling apart!

⭐ **Give them permission to leave:** Seriously, tell them verbally, they can leave when they're ready!

FIVE STAGES OF GRIEF ~ *Elisabeth Kübler-Ross*

It is helpful to understand the grieving process of any loss in life. Everyone needs to go through this experience in his or her own way, for as long as it takes. Don't try to buffer someone's encounter with grief. Be there for support and encouragement, but give them the space to work through the process themselves. I spent my life running interference for everyone. God said to me on more than one occasion, "I'm trying to work here and you're in my way by continually running interference for everyone! Move over!" I thought it was my job to "protect" everyone! I didn't want anyone to suffer, so I would "protect" and *absorb their pain.* By doing this, I prevented their growth and prolonged lessons that the soul had come to learn.

Once again, by letting others have their life experiences, you allow them an opportunity for growth and you let them experience their own personal power.

Not everyone experiences all of the stages of grief, and often people will vacillate back and forth between several stages. It is important that no one be rushed through the grieving process. It is an individual journey, and everyone has his or her own way of processing.

It is in the pain that we learn; it is working
though the pain that we heal.

Denial ~ "I feel fine." "This can't be happening, not to me." Denial is usually only a temporary defense for the individual. This feeling is generally replaced with heightened awareness of situations and individuals that will be left behind after death.

Anger ~ "Why me?" "It's not fair!" "Who is to blame?" Once in the second stage, the individual recognizes that denial cannot continue. Because of anger, the person is difficult to care for due to misplaced feelings of rage and envy. Any individual who symbolizes life or energy is subject to projected resentment and jealousy.

Bargaining ~ "Just let me live to see my children graduate." "I'll do anything for a few more years." "I'll give my life savings if…" The third stage involves the hope that the individual can somehow postpone or delay death. Usually, the negotiation for an extended life is made with a higher power in exchange for a reformed lifestyle. Psychologically, the person is saying, "I understand I will die, but if I could just have more time..."

Depression ~ "It's so sad, why bother with anything?" "I'm going to die...what's the point?" "I miss my loved one, why go on?" During the fourth stage, the dying person begins to understand the certainty of death. Because of this, the individual may become silent, refuse visitors, and spend much of the time crying and grieving. This process allows the dying person to disconnect himself or herself from things of love and affection. It is not recommended to attempt to cheer up an individual who is in this stage. It is an important time for grieving that must be processed.

Accept ~ "It's going to be okay." "I can't fight it, so I may as well prepare for it." This final stage comes with peace and understanding of the death that is approaching. Generally, the person in the fifth stage will want to be left alone. Additionally, feelings and physical pain may be non-existent. This stage has also been described as the end of the dying struggle.

Chapter 7

SPIRITUAL COACHING AND SOUL RESCUING

MY CALLING AS A DOULA AND SOUL RESCUER, WITH A SLIGHT TWIST

The word *doula* came to me one day in meditation. I didn't actually know its meaning, so I went to the trusty dictionary, which defined *doula* as "A woman experienced in childbirth who provides advice, information, and emotional support to a mother, infant, and family, before, during, and just after childbirth."

That is absolutely what I have done in my life! I've been a doula, not only to babies, my own as well as others, but to dogs, cats, and ponies! Now, however, it has expanded to providing support for the birthing into the next life as well. I have been led to people and places where an opportunity has opened up and I have felt *called*. Sometimes a soul may have become confused because of an accident and has trouble with the transitioning to the *after life*. I ask for guidance and support on their behalf from the Spirit World Ascended Masters (holy men and women who are in heaven), including Jesus, Mary, saints, guardian angels, and ancestors. I become an open channel for *Divine Energy* and *Guidance* for the soul needing support. This is also what I do when I practice *Energy Healing* work; I simply allow myself to become an open channel for *Divine Energy* to heal.

> *Just as we employ midwives to help an infant in its birth, we would be wise in this culture to employ individuals specially trained to help us die.*
>
> ~ Ram Dass, *Still Here*

SPIRITUAL COACHING

We are not the predictors of when the transition will take place—we are simply called to hold sacred space for those in transition, to listen to what they want, what they want to talk about, and share our experience. It's that simple!

I learned this lesson the hard way. I made the mistake of opening my mouth as I went to help my friend's mother in Ireland, while he was doing some remodeling to her house. When I arrived, he said to me, "I need my mother to live for ten more years." After seeing her, I said, "She may decide to leave after Christmas." I later was sorry that I had made such a remark, as it had affected him deeply. I had been taking notes about her health, and it was clear to me, when I read back, that she was much less healthy, mentally and physically, when I first arrived. I returned home from a night away and my friend said, "She's looking great, you're doing a great job with her. She doesn't look like a woman who will be dead by Christmas." I was horrified to hear my words reflected back to me. I apologized and acknowledged, "No one knows." It's simply up to God and the person in transition. Needless to say, I will not make that mistake ever again!

The following steps are the things I do when I'm spending time with a person going through end-of-life transition:

Before I Arrive

⭐ I pray before I arrive at each encounter. In gratitude, I give thanks for the opportunity, ask for support, and invite any help—anyone from the Light (angels, saints, ancestors, etc.) who wish to be present and help with the work we're assisting with for the highest good of all, harming none.

⭐ When time permits, I practice some kind of moving meditation, usually Sheng Zhen Qigong. Collecting positive energy, I then consciously and visually ground to the earth and connect to heaven, becoming an open channel for divine energy flow.

While I'm There

⭐ I talk with family and friends, taking in their insights and concerns.

⭐ I don't push my agenda. I wait patiently for the correct opening. I let the person I'm visiting take the lead.

⭐ I get on their playing field. I use language that is comforting to them. I become a part of their world—eating, drinking tea, whatever makes them feel comfortable. I accept them as they are and I don't try to change them in any way. I meet them where they are and I move forward with caution and gentleness, always asking and watching for higher guidance.

⭐ The entire time that I am with them, I watch and listen to their reactions, words, and body language, and their openness or resistance to what I am saying. When something isn't getting a positive and open response, I move in another direction. In asking for spiritual direction, I listen to my heart, and I pay attention for clues, as to what to do next.

I trust that they will get what they need, perhaps by osmosis. It's not my business what they appear to *get* or *not get*. It's simply my assignment to be present: holding sacred space, sharing experiences, and listening to anything they want to say. Their words provide a treasure map of what needs to be healed. Usually, love for themselves, trusting God and themselves, and letting go and receiving are the three main things that come up over and over.

I find that it is very important to touch the person in transition. They perhaps can't accept a hug, but maybe a gentle, hand, head, or foot massage. Many times I will rub their feet and toes while I am talking with them. I simply follow my inner guidance to know what I should do.

I continually offer encouragement, saying only positive things, especially about them. Sometimes negative messages they've been carrying around about themselves get in the way of their feeling worthy, which hinders their ability to peacefully let go of their body. If they don't trust that they will go to heaven, I will tell them that everyone has a skeleton in the closet, something they think will keep them from going to heaven, but it's simply not true.

Before I Leave

⭐ I offer a prayer out loud while doing a head massage. I pray very gently, lovingly, and slowly, addressing and releasing any concerns they shared with me in our visit, restating everything in a positive manner. I end by asking for their guardian angel and St. Michael to come and protect them, their property, their house, and their families. Then I explain that it is important that they trust that it will be so. If they hear a bump in the night or feel uneasy, I advise them to breathe deeply and relax while thanking St. Michael for protecting them.

When I Leave

⭐ As I leave I offer some pointers for them to consider. It may be that they begin to think about turning around their negative feelings. Also, if they can't think of something grand to say about themselves, I do it for them. I touch them, in a way that is nurturing, maybe on the shoulder or hand.

Bits and Pieces

⭐ A shaman told me that lighting eight candles calls for the ancestors.

⭐ I play a song called "Calling All Angels" (from the *Pay*

It Forward soundtrack*)*, which gathers the angels to the sacred space.

In Tibetan practice, for example, monks and nuns are instructed in ways to guide the dying through their transition. They are trained to deal with the dying person's thirst, coldness, heaviness, and breathlessness, encouraging the one who is dying not to cling to these phenomena. They offer such instructions as these: "As the earth element leaves, your body will feel heavy. As the water element leaves, you will feel dryness. As the fire element leaves, you may feel cold. As the air element leaves, your out breath will be longer than your in breath. The signs are now here. Don't get lost in the detail. Don't cling to any of these phenomena. They are part of a natural process. Let your Awareness go free.

~ Ram Dass, *Still Here*

In the Hawaiian spiritual tradition, the breath is very sacred. It is given to family members or someone considered *family* as a greeting. It is considered a sacred gift to receive the last breath of someone who is dying, and this ritual is done in a very conscious way. The question was put to a Hawaiian Shaman, "How can you time the last breath transfer?" His reply was, "It can be given at any time when the transition nears and often death is soon after the transfer of the HA breath. It is different than the Hawaiian greeting in that it is often accompanied by visions. It can also occur in Dreamtime as was the case with my father. I received the HA breath while asleep on the mainland."

Truthfully, you don't need any real formula or ritual for helping souls to cross over. You will discover your own way. All you need is the intention. Energy follows intention. We are energy: The intention is for a safe and peaceful crossing over to the next life! It's that simple!

HELP FOR THE FINAL TRANSITION (LEAVING THE BODY)

Helping with the final transition is sometimes very hard for the family to do, as they are too close to the person. It may be hard for the one in transition to receive from the family as well. It doesn't matter who this tenderness comes from.

Care for the one in transition as you would care for a young child as you're putting them to bed.

1. Tell them a story: what to expect, what's going to happen, and that they will have visitors to escort them safely across to the other side, towards the Light.

2. Touch, massage, and kiss them. *Let them hold your*

hand, which is different than you holding theirs. Rub their feet and toes. This touching calms and relaxes them. It's a key component.

3. Tell them how important they are and that you love them.

4. Tell them everything is going to be fine with who and what they are leaving behind.

5. Tell them that it is safe for them to leave whenever they are ready.

6. Tell them that we are all going to heaven. Nothing they have done will keep this gift from them.

The soul needs time to transition

I learned this firsthand from my mother. I didn't know about giving the soul time to adjust when I was taking care of her. My mother died, and I had her whisked away. I got her room cleaned up straight away! Within a few hours, you'd never have known that my mother had been present in my home at all. A week passed and I got a phone call from my brother in Missouri. He began, "I don't think Mom has left yet!" "What do you mean? She's not here!" I exclaimed! He continued, "I saw Sandy (our sister who had made the transition several years prior) in heaven instantly, but I haven't seen Mom yet. I think she's still at your house!" This was all new for me. I was working at a church with a 150-year-old school on the premises. The handyman from church was always telling me about *presences* he felt on the third floor! I told him what my brother had said and asked him if he would go to my house and see what he thought. He came back with the announcement that he felt a presence near my desk in the family room (exactly where my mom's bed had been.) My friend prayed and told her to seek the Light. It was time to move on. He checked a few days later, and she had left.

My dad, on the other hand, had all the time he needed to transition. After the experience with my mom, I knew his soul needed time. My prayer had been, "Thank you that when the time came my dad's body would remain where it was, as long as was needed for his transition." As it happened, his body remained at his home for over five hours. The mortuary apologized for how long it took to pick the body up; it was unusual that it would take so long. But I just smiled because I knew it was how long his soul needed for the transition.

In my grandparents' time, in the Midwest, the body was laid out at home for a week, with plenty of time for the soul to transition, plenty of time for the ones left behind to make peace.

While I was staying in Ireland, the father of an acquaintance died unexpectedly. He told me about his father's wake. They laid out his dad at their family home for a day—the length of time depends on how long it takes the whole family to make it home. Family, friends, and community come by to pay their respects, eat, and drink. Some of the family members take turns spending the night with the corpse so it is never left unattended. It is a very touching custom and it gives everyone the space to heal and release.

TWO STORIES OF PEOPLE I'VE BEEN LEAD TO

The following short stories were written about my first real knowledge that I was chosen to assist another in transitioning from this life.

My Friend Joe

Joe has been a friend of mine since I was a secretary at our local parish. He was a parishioner and my son's best friend's grandpa. Joe was the pastor's right-hand man when it came to volunteering and fixing things around the church grounds. Joe and I had a special *soul* connection, maybe because he reminded me of my dad who lived far away.

My last visit with Joe was a couple of months before he passed. I noticed he was getting tired and his appetite had left. That was the last time I saw Joe before a feeling of *needing* to pay him a visit kept nagging at me. (Maybe it was a gentle nudging from his guardian angel!)

I arrived and asked to see Joe. His daughter smiled and hesitantly said, "I don't know if he'll know you." I replied, "Well then, can I come in and say hi to Helen (his wife)?" I walked through the opening into the family room where Joe was lying in a hospital bed. He had oxygen on and Helen was sitting next to him holding his hand. I began to cry and asked Helen how she was doing. She smiled, as she always did, and replied "Fine." I leaned over and whispered to her, "But it sure doesn't feel fine sometimes, does it?"

I went over to Joe and began in my usual lighthearted way, "Hey Joe, I heard the cutest boy in town lived here and I just wanted to come and see for myself!" I then took his hand, stroked his arm, and began in a more serious manner to tell him some things I wanted to say: "Joe, we had some fabulous times. I could always talk you into letting me help you do stuff nobody else would let me do. Remember when you let me climb to the top of the church, and then you called up to me, 'Pati, come down, I'm not feeling so good!' You really gave me a scare! I love you, Joe." I thanked him for the great times we shared together and then I said I needed to get back to work. (Well, that wasn't so hard!)

I turned my attention to Helen. "It was my experience with my mom that they can hear you all the way to the end, even when you think they can't." I walked over to Joe and once again took his hand, stroked it, and began speaking of spiritual matters. I said, "Joe, I know you hear me, I can feel you squeezing my hand," and he squeezed it harder.

They had just finished saying a rosary, and that's exactly what I would have done in my previous experiences with the dying. Praying was all I was taught in my Christian life. Prayer in any form is comforting to most people. Now, I have been able to see that there are many other tools that can also be used for comfort and the safe journey home.

"He's afraid to die," his daughter confided in me. I told her, "That's been my experience with the people I've been with before. It seems that they reflect back on their lives and they see God as a scorekeeper and, of course, no one measures up. The fear of not making it to heaven feels very real, and the question arises, "If I'm not good enough for God, well then, who *am* I good enough for, and where will I end up?" (Concept adapted from author Terry Hershey.)

I continued stroking Joe's hand. "Joe you've left quite a legacy here on this earth. You've learned your lessons well, and you need not worry about anything; everyone is going to be just fine. You've provided well for your family. Helen, your children, your grandchildren and great grandchildren, they are all going to be just fine. You've done a fantastic job!"

I looked into his eyes, and I said, "Joe, baby, what I know is this. We have a loving, forgiving, compassionate, and merciful God. I think this life is about experiencing love, joy, and peace, as well as about learning. The mistakes we think we've made in our life, well, they're just that. They are simply mistakes. It's how we learn. It's the questions we get wrong on the tests that we remember! The Bible says, "It is not the wish of my Father that anyone be lost," and "In My Father's house there are many rooms and I go before you to prepare one for you, if this were not so, I could not be telling you." Isn't God fabulous? Look at these words of comfort that God has given to us.

Joe, let me tell you a little story. It begins with Jesus speaking. "Joe, I love you simply because I love you. You were made in the likeness and image of God, how could it be any different? You can do nothing to earn my love. It's purely a grace. When you get to the gates of heaven, Joe, I'll be waiting for you, and I'll say 'Joe, I'm delighted you're here.' I'll go and get that Big Book, you know, the one that we keep with all of the names of the people who will be coming home, and I'll read everything that is written about you. It simply says...Joe. I may even read it a couple of times, Joe... Joe. Because you see, Joe, that's all there is in the Big Book. The things that you did that were good—I didn't count them, I simply enjoyed it when you did them. The mistakes you think you made? Well, I didn't count them either. They are simply how you learn. You see, that is why I died on the cross. Then I'll take you in and introduce you to My Father and He'll wink at you and say, 'That's some Joe ya got there, Jesus,' and all the angels and saints will celebrate, and you'll come and plop yourself down next to Me on My big white throne and we'll have us a big practice laugh before we really get this party started. Then My Father will turn to you and say, 'This is My son Joe, in whom I am well pleased.'"

I continued with, "Joe baby, we're going to miss you and the tears we are crying are for ourselves. When you're ready, honey, you simply let go and follow the Light. Your spirit will be free to fly." As I left, I gave him a final kiss on the forehead and stroked his arm all the way down to his hand, which I took and pressed against the one lone tear on my cheek. Then with one final kiss, I said with the biggest smile in my heart and on my face, "Hey Joe, I'll catch you on the flip side," and with that, I left.

As I drove back to work, an old familiar tune by Kenny Loggins took over my mind… *Please, Celebrate me Home!* Joe left for his new home early the next morning.

George

I went to visit a man named George—not a visit I had planned to make. His son, Brad, had told me that his father wanted to die, and it just happened that I found myself in his home while waiting for a ride.

I sat at the table while George ate his dinner, and we spoke frankly about his wanting to die. I began in a lighthearted way by asking him if he'd like to dance, even though he was using a walker! He said with a gentle smile, "Maybe next week!" I asked him what he would miss when it was his time to go. I told him that he could choose when he wanted to leave this earth. He looked pretty darn healthy to me, and I personally thought that he should work on living rather than dying. I shared with him my dad's experience, and that

I believed that he had some say in when he was ready to leave this earth

After dinner George went to bed. I went and tucked him in. I began asking him questions about what he wanted and if he was afraid. I said good night and went back to the table, where a family member told me that George had been a gay man who married, had four children, and then divorced. I knew instantly that George had some guilt that would keep him here on this earth longer than necessary if he didn't get these feelings of failure resolved. I went back to George's room, much to his son's dismay, but I didn't speak of anything personal. I only knew he needed to know that he too was going to heaven. I asked him if he believed in a Higher Power. His son told me he didn't believe in God. But when I asked him, he said yes. I told George that we are on this earth to learn. The things we do in our lives are simply how we learn; the mistakes we make—or think we make—are just how we learn. God is not looking to keep us from Him. God does not keep a score card, marking all the bad things we *think* we've done. We were created in the likeness and image of God, so why would God try to keep us from Himself?

I took his head in my hands, kissed him on his forehead, on each cheek, and then on the lips. "I love you, George. Now you rest." I went to the kitchen where I could see that Brad was upset. Brad knew that his dad wanted to die, but before my visit it had just been words; now it was taking on a reality of its own. "The only thing I can tell you, Brad, is that I had no intention of coming here to your house and yet here I stand. I need to do what it feels like I'm here to do. Now, your father may choose to leave when you're not here. Don't fret about it. George knows what he is doing. Sometimes they do not want the family around when they transition out."

Several months later, while in Ireland, I received an email from Brad's girlfriend.

Hello Pati,
Brad and I are doing well. Much has happened since your visit to George's house. George died at the end of August on a Friday night. It was a very beautiful and moving moment. I have never been present or in the same house to witness someone's death.

TWO STORIES OF PLACES I'VE BEEN LED TO FOR *SOUL RESCUING*

My calling to begin soul rescuing began in a session with my spiritual director several years ago. It was suggested to me that I begin visiting cemeteries, just to be present and to pray. For what, I wondered. I didn't know. As I began traveling around the world, I made it a point to visit any place I felt like I should see. My first experience was in Hawaii at a cemetery next to an old Catholic church by the sea. After mass, I walked through the cemetery and read tombstones. I began praying for anyone who needed assistance. I asked St. Michael to come for protection, and then I invited them to seek the Light. I asked for my guardian angels and ancestors to find their guardian angels and ancestors to help with the escorting to the Light. I had no idea if it was right. I just followed my instincts.

A couple of years later, while on an extended stay in Ireland, there had been an accident on an island called Skelligs Michael. Skelligs is a rock island, 715 feet high, and eight miles off the coast of Kerry. It is lined with stone stairs with no railings or shrubs that stretch all the way to the top of this magnificent rock. In the early 1800s, it had been the center of monastic life for the Irish Christian monks. The victim was a woman visiting the island from New York who had slipped off the path and fell to her death.

I knew I wanted to go to Skelligs, but I wasn't sure exactly why. Was it to experience the monastery and the views, or was it because of the accident, or was it something about the monastery itself? The Irish people I was staying with told me it was too dangerous and that I shouldn't go. But I knew I was going, and it wasn't out of defiance (which can be the case with me) but rather because I knew I had to go. I was able to talk an Irish friend into accompanying me.

The sea was very rough on the hour-long boat ride over to the island. I found that I began introducing myself to the sea. (This was something that I had learned from the Hawaiian Spiritual Tradition while in Hawaii. It is my understanding that they believe that all Spirit comes from the water. You start by introducing yourself to the ocean, and then you ask for protection from the ocean—a place that deserves the utmost respect.) I noticed myself in a very aware state after I said these words: "Thank you for protecting us while we are on our way to the island for the work that I'm about to do." I thought I was going for a spiritual purpose, but after the words left my mouth, I became aware of the fact that I was truly going to work to do some soul rescuing.

All day during the climb upward, and especially at the top around the monastery, I performed the same ritual I had been doing in other cemeteries I'd been visiting. I prayed in gratitude, gave thanks, and asked for help and guidance. On our hike up the mountain, I wasn't able to see where the woman had slipped off of the path, but I knew there had been a potted flower set at the place where she fell. It wasn't until on the way down, when my friend and I reached the bottom of the stairs, that we turned the corner and found the flowers. What else could I do but ask her (in a spiritual sense) if she needed help? I explained to her that she had an accident and that her body was no

longer available to her. We talked, and I asked for support
and guidance for her.

Then I had to trust that the reason for my wanting to
go to Skelligs had been fulfilled.

Mary

A few months later, still in Ireland, I woke up
with these words fresh in my mind: "Go to the
beach!" *What? Why? Which beach? And do what?
Take a walk? Commune with nature?* The thought
quickly left my mind, and a bit later my friend's
sister-in-law called and asked if I would go to the
neighborhood village to pick up some meat for
her. I was happy to do it. As it turned out, I didn't
know how to get there at all! I began by turning
right out the driveway and found myself driving
along the coastline. I remember thinking, *Ah,
the beach!* I drove for a bit, and then a bit longer,
thinking, *This can't be right.* So I drove to a nearby
cluster of houses, turned around, and drove back. I
noticed a road sign that said "Clare Strand." I knew
that a *strand* was a beach, so I stopped and called
home on my cell phone to say that I was lost and
I'd be a bit later in returning. In the meantime I
thought, *Pretty tricky way to get me to go to the
beach!* I drove down the road to the strand. During
my time in Ireland, my eighty-year-old friend

Martha had told me many times the story of her friend who had drowned in the sea when they were both thirteen. I couldn't remember her name, but suddenly *Mary* came into my awareness. "Oh, Mary honey, is it you? Do you need help in crossing over?" I stopped at the beach which was at the end of the road and began praying. I called upon St. Michael to come for protection. Then I invited anyone from the Light to come and assist us. Next, I asked for my guardian angels and ancestors to contact her guardian angels and ancestors to assist us in showing her the way home. I began to talk with her, "Mary, honey, I'm so sorry. You've had an accident and your body is no longer available to you. It is safe for you to follow your guardian angels and ancestors to the Light. You're free to leave now, sweetheart, just go with your loved ones. Go to the Light."

Once again, it occurred to me that when a person dies suddenly, the soul can sometimes become confused. I also know the soul knows no time. So while this accident took place many years ago in actual earth time, it could appear to be the same day to this little girl. I began to smile inside while standing there on the strand. I openly said, "No," I wasn't going to the beach. I didn't understand, and yet there I was, with the persistence and guidance of the Spirit World. I then turned to the little cemetery on the side of the road overlooking the sea, the place where Martha said all the babies who washed up from the sea were buried. Although this never really made sense to me, she talked about this cemetery often as well. Was it a place where un-baptized babies were buried? Nevertheless, finding myself standing in front of this cemetery, would I dare say "No" again because I didn't understand? Not a chance! So I did the same ritual for any of the souls in the cemetery that had not been able to find their way home. I always end with a prayer of love and gratitude for being chosen to be a part of someone's journey; for being still enough to listen; for the support I receive, even when I'm not fully tuned in, like this day when "Go to the beach!" was whispered in my ear. (An added note: Martha never told me the story of her young friend Mary or the babies in the cemetery again. Was it because they were finally free?)

AN ADDED NOTE ~ HEALING FOR SOULS WHO CROSS OUR PATH

While I am driving along roads and highways, and crosses with ribbons, flowers, and other tokens of love and remembrances enter my awareness, I am prompted to pray. I ask for assistance for any souls who may have been confused about their accident, speaking to them just as I did with Mary.

I share these experiences with you because they are not just my experiences. I am just a person who is open and willing to be used. We are all called. I'm sure you will recognize similar situations in your own life when you're paying attention and know what you're looking for.

★

More recently, I had been to the market several times trying to get money from Western Union.

It was interesting to me how hard it was to get this money. Customer service was closed, then the money hadn't been sent correctly, then they didn't have any money to cash the check. Finally, after five tries, the money was finally available, and I happened to notice a lady in line behind me who looked like she needed a hug. (This wouldn't have happened had the money been available earlier ☺.) I asked her if it would be okay if I gave her one. She seemed appreciative and explained that her adult son had died six months earlier. I told her that I was writing a book that she might be interested in, so I got her phone number.

★

The next day, I was doing some healing work on a client when this woman's son came to my mind. A light bulb went on and I knew her son (his soul) hadn't been free to leave this realm. Even though it had been six months, his mother hadn't been able to let go yet. She was still wearing his dog tags around her neck, and her bedroom had been transformed into a shrine for him. I called her and asked her if she had time to meet for tea. She felt safe to tell her story, and then I told her of my calling as a *soul rescuer.* I told her that I felt her son was stuck because she couldn't let go. She acknowledged that what I was saying was correct. Sitting at a table in front of the market, we did a *sending off ritual*, asking for protection and guidance for her son's safe crossing to the next life. The mother said all the things that she never got to say to her son because of his sudden death, and she acknowledged that she was preventing them both from moving on. Not only did I feel him leaving, but the mother did also. I gave her a homework assignment to reclaim her bedroom by packing all of her son's items away, including the dog tags, and to make her bedroom fresh and lovely for herself. It's not that we forget the person who's passed; it's that we love them enough to set them free! When I left, she had a new light in her eyes.

Chapter 8

COMFORT FOR THOSE LEFT BEHIND

PRACTICAL HELP TO BEGIN THE HEALING PROCESS

Give Yourself Permission and Time to Heal

After the loss of my dad, I hated the consolation words, the patronizing phrases, "I'm sorry for your loss," or "Thank you for taking care of your dad!" Why would other people be thanking me for taking care of my father? It's not easy, of course, to provide words of comfort for a person who's experiencing the transition of a loved one. I can't think of any examples of things people said to me that were comforting.

While it's different for everyone, all I wanted was to be left alone! I just needed time to be with the emptiness, the pain, and the transition for myself. I told a friend, "I feel funky." I couldn't think. I had no direction. I didn't know what to do. My friend's wise words helped me get some clarity. "Pati, you've spent all your time, focus, and energy for the past months caring for one person, and now suddenly he's gone. You will need time to heal to know what to do with your time and the void that is left." I related it to planning a wedding. A person may spend months, even years, planning for one special day, and when it's over, it's over! Now what? What will define your days? All of your attention and energy now has no place to go.

I'd been busy for so long that it seemed novel to me to just *be*. It felt foreign. I felt guilty for being *lazy* and *wasting time*. After my dad died, a friend of mine stopped over, and I was lying on the couch. He asked me if I was sick. I said no, but actually, I was sick. I was exhausted—physically and emotionally!

Being on overdrive for so many months had taken its toll on my well-being. I had no choice but to stop, rest, and redefine how I would spend my days and regain control of life again. It took time; a lot of time, rest, hot baths, massage, and much more than I could than have imagined to help revive myself.

A dear friend has brought this point up to me many times and I have just kind of ignored it. However, during the final edits of this book, she called to tell me again, so I'll pass on this information here.

She began, "I never saw anything like it! When you

were finished taking care of your father, a piece of you had died as well. You looked like something the cat had drug in. It took over a year of recovery: body work, massage, therapy, and resting for you to begin healing. You were so very tired. I have never seen you look like that! Tell your readers how you got through it and stayed intact. How did you pull yourself back to the living?"

The only thing I remember about this time in my life was that not only had I lost my father (physically), I had lost the purpose of my life, or so it felt like. For the last six months, my dad was my total focus. He was a great diversion to place my personal journey on hold.

I was also the executor of my dad's estate. I had the added responsibilities (and graces) of cleaning up my dad's physical assets and investing them for the beneficiaries. Maybe in the old days, the *mourning period* was a year-long for a reason—a time when nothing was expected from you.

Give yourself as much time as you need without making any excuses. Do whatever feels right to you, and if that means staying in bed for awhile or not answering the phone, well, then do it!

The movie *P.S. I Love You* is a wonderful example of how this beginning mourning can look. A young woman looses her husband to an illness and needs some time and space to process what has happened in her life. Her family and friends, well intended, try to get her to move through her process faster than she is ready, but she sticks to her guns and takes all the time she needs.

I can't really give feedback on how to heal from a loved one dying; I can only share with you what I know. I promise you, there is a glorious life awaiting you at the end of it all!

> *Take all the time and space you need . . .*
> *for YOU!*

STAYING SAD IS A HINDERANCE TO EVERYONE

While I was in massage school, there was a book in the library written by someone who claimed to have channeled messages from John Lennon after his death, which caught my eye. One of the things I found intriguing was what this author reported that Lennon had said about people grieving for him. "I am happy and peaceful where I am. I feel your pain. I try to absorb it and transform it to positive energy and send it back to you, but you have to learn to do this for yourself."

Our feeling sorry or guilty will not bring people back to life. In fact, it is a hindrance to them where they are. The best thing we can do is to go through our own grieving process, acknowledging our loss, and then move on. We don't forget them; we remember them with light and love. They want us to be happy, too.

Let yourself grieve, feel the loss, be depressed.

Sleep as much as you need. Our bodies heal from resting.

Talk about it—your memories, your anger—talk some more.

Cry about it, cry some more.

Don't feel like you've abandoned them if you move forward.

Remember your pain causes them pain.

Remember they are happy.

They want to be a support from the other side. Pay attention: Watch, ask.

LEARNING TO READ THE SUPPORT AND SIGNS FROM NATURE

I touched on this in an earlier part of the book, but it was so important to me when my dad transitioned to the next life that I think it needs a section here as well.

These little stories about some of my experiences with my dad are just examples of how we can *see* the support of *God and the Spirit World* in everything. All we have to do is be still, watch, listen, and feel.

I arrived at the Denver airport for my flight home from Missouri just after finding out that my dad was dying. I decided to call him from the airport. It was difficult to hold back the tears, but I wanted him to know that I supported and respected however he wanted to live out the rest of his life here on earth. I told him, "I admire that you want to *live* the rest of your life and not just *exist*, Dad. I appreciate the fact that you do not want to end your days taking pills and being hooked up to a dialysis machine." After I hung up, I decided that I would write him a letter affirming his successes and achievements—something I hadn't done enough. I told him how I felt I hadn't been able to help my mom exactly how I would have liked to at the time she was dying, and how I would maybe do better this time. I would come to him if he didn't want to come to California.

As I was waiting for my flight, I saw the most incredible, vibrant rainbow—all colors: purple, blue, green, yellow, orange, red; bright and crystal clear. I knew it was a sign that no matter what happened, it was all going to be okay. It was all good. It was simply Divine Order.

A week later I was in Chicago, sitting at the lake's edge in the courtyard of a church, when out of the clear blue came a short shower with huge raindrops. I knew that these were tears from the angels for my dad. Once again, they were a reassurance to me that everything was happening in Divine Order.

After my dad passed, my flight attendant daughter relayed her experience of her Papa's dying to me. She received the call of her Papa's passing while away on a trip. She told me that on her break, she looked out the plane window and asked her Papa to send her a shooting star; he sent five! She was very touched. (The number five means *change*.)

At my dad's memorial, I read a paper I had written entitled, "He Did It His Way." Later, all four of my adult children asked me at different times, what *Hummingbird Medicine* meant. "Joy," I told them. As it turned out, there had been a hummingbird flying around behind me the whole time I was reading. This was very touching to all of us, as hummingbirds had been a huge love of my dad's.

And then, while looking for answers and trying to make sense out of my dad's dying, I began paying attention. There were many other signs from my dad as I was settling his estate. Support often came in the form of hummingbirds. From the very big decision to sell his home in Missouri to the last property I sold in California, there were always hummingbirds present. One day, while trying to decide about selling his Missouri home, I went to one of his flowerbeds to pull weeds, think, and pray. I noticed a beautiful Iris plant in full bloom when a hummingbird came to collect some nectar. Two days later the same iris plant was completely withered and dry, completely closed up. I knew it was a message that I could let this place go. It once was alive; now it was finished. I sold the house.

While I was in Ireland, a friend's father unexpectedly passed. We were standing outside when my friend looked up and said, "See that star? That's the first thing I saw the night my dad passed. For me, that's exactly where he is." I later found out it was the planet Jupiter, the planet of opportunity, blessings, expansion beyond normal bounds, optimism, and luck. (The luck of the Irish!) Wow, what a great place to begin one's journey home!

Our loved ones are always with us. They want us to remember. They want to help us with our life's journey. All we have to do is pay attention to the signs they're sending. Pay attention to songs that play on the radio, commercials on TV, nature, animals that cross your path, the wind chimes tinkling in the wind. These are the things that our loved ones and the angels use to try and get our attention. Guidance and signs are everywhere!

> *Pay attention to what you see! Know that your intuition is right!*

> *The first thing that comes to your mind is your answer!*

WHO WILL YOU BE WHEN YOU REALIZE YOU AREN'T WHO YOU THOUGHT YOU WERE?

When all of your attention and time isn't tied up with the life of another, you will be free to focus on you—to do your personal work and take care of yourself. Sometimes the easy part is focusing on others, being a caregiver to a parent or loved one, being a mother and focusing on your children, or simply focusing on other people or your job. Being a workaholic is one addiction that is accepted and sometimes even admired in our society! But in fact it's about *doing* to the excess. We may not even notice, but *as long as I'm focused on something else, it keeps my focus off of me!* Some may get lost in their iPods, cell phones, or computers. Anything we do in excess, anything that keeps us from being with ourselves, anything that prevents us from knowing who we are, can manifest as an addiction— the emotional work has been stuffed.

I remember years ago saying to someone, "I don't really know who I am. I don't want to know, I don't want others to know. If they did, they may not like me. Heck, *I* may not like me!"

In the movie *As Good As it Gets,* the young mother played by Helen Hunt spends every spare second worrying about her asthmatic son. When someone comes along to help her, she doesn't know how to act. As her son's health improves, she suddenly has spare time on her hands with no one to worry about, and she notices how lonely she is. What is a person to do when confronted by such a hard truth? Spending all your time taking care of someone or something else, becomes a wonderful diversion from taking care of yourself.

> *By living in the moment there are no regrets, fears, anticipation or anxieties.*
>
> *It's only about this moment and it is never not . . . this moment. Peace will follow.*
> ~ Eckhart Tolle, *The Power of Now*

FOOD FOR THOUGHT

⭐ Sometimes you have to let go of your desires for the happiness of another.

⭐ Remember…it is all about LOVE.

⭐ You have to go through the anger and pain—feel it, experience it—before healing can begin.

⭐ Give yourself permission to heal, rest, scream, cry, yell.

⭐ Take time to *just be*—be alone, grieve your loss.

⭐ Transform your pain or you may transfer your pain to others.

⭐ You can become bitter or better—the choice is up to you.

⭐ Write—journaling will help you sort out your feelings.

⭐ Let the tears flow—write through them, ask them what they are about.

⭐ There is no *quick fix*, no pill that will take the place of the inward journey.

⭐ After your journey through the desert you will see from a new vantage point.

⭐ Let go of any guilt you may be carrying.

⭐ Forgive yourself first; then you can forgive others.

⭐ Remember we have a merciful and loving Creator, not a scorekeeping God.

⭐ In our pain, religion can take a back seat to spirituality (these are two different things).

⭐ Intense pain can ultimately become an opening to a spiritual awakening.

⭐ Remember that all things are in Divine Order.

⭐ Trust that God knows what He is doing and has a plan.

⭐ Let go of your expectations—how you think things should be—and accept how they are.

⭐ Say *yes* to what shows up in your life.

> *True Freedom comes when we are detached from anything of this world.*
> ~ Author Unknown

> *It's not that we fear death,*
> *It's that we fear we come to the end of our lives*
> *And realize that we never really lived!*
> ~ Author Unknown

TIDBITS

⭐ I believe that we are, at times, co-creators with God, and that we have some say in when we leave this earth. I believe that when the soul is finished with whatever it is here to do in this life, it is free to leave. My dad absolutely chose when he was leaving as we all watched.

⭐ We all have a valid place on the wheel of life. We all have our gifts, even when others live their lives differently than we do. We all have talents to share, and we're all just here learning our lessons, just like everyone else (as different as we all may be)!

It's important that we have compassion for everyone, especially ourselves. We need to be aware that we are all products of our past—including our childhoods, generations past and present, and the cultures in which we were raised.

Appendix

TIPS FOR THE ONE IN TRANSITION

THE POINT OF NO RETURN: WHEN YOU REALIZE THAT YOUR DAYS ARE NUMBERED

> *"Do not fear...I have called you by name: you are Mine!"*
>
> ~ Isaiah 43:1

You've gotten the news. It's terminal. There's no hope for recovery, or maybe you're simply getting on in years. It's then that you've reached the point of "No Return." You already know it intellectually; it's inevitable. It's when you begin to feel it in your heart, and when you realize there are no *bargaining tools* left in the bag, when you can't say, "Stop! I've changed my mind, let me off this ride!" It's when you have no control over what was familiar; when you know there's nothing left to do but simply wait and wait some more, knowing full well—the final outcome— Curtains! It's like a Ferris wheel ride. You hop on the ride at birth and you ride the wheel for the cycle of your life. You reach the top and then it begins to come down. You have to get off, there are no other options; you can't go around again. The time has come. It's then that we must learn to surrender, walk, sit, or lie down for our final days on this earth with a clear knowing and a trust that our God is in control. It's not up to you any longer when you reach this point. He'll drive the car that will get us home safely. It's a complete and total trusting and surrendering.

> *I will never forget you, I hold you in the palm of my hand.*
>
> ~ Isaiah 11

WHERE WILL I END UP?

Whether you're just getting on in years or you've been diagnosed with an illness, you know your days are limited and that it's time to say good-bye to this earth and all that you love. Now is a good time to reminisce back through your life, to take a journey down memory lane. My experience is that everyone begins to wonder and ask themselves a few questions around this point in time. What was it all about? What difference did I make? What mistakes did I make? What did I participate in or allow? If you've come from a strict religious upbringing and your God is the same God you had in your youth, you haven't given Him the space to expand; it could be that you have a pretty conservative, even toxic, perception of God. If you perceive God as scorekeeper, then you might be thinking: *If I'm not good enough for God, who am I good enough for and where will I end up?*

It's at this point that you need to be kind to *you!* You were made in the likeness and image of God. He has no scorecard. He simply has the Book of Life and *you,* my friend, are in it! You are loved because you are a child of God. It's a grace. *You are going to heaven!* Now rest in that, trust in God, and when the little voices in your head begin to tell you otherwise, be firm. Thank them for coming, but then send them on their way with their little backpacks of negative talk in tow! Replace any negative thoughts with loving affirmations of how God loves and cares for you each and every moment.

You're already a living prayer, God hears you as you breathe.
~ Author Unknown

THE FINAL LESSONS BEFORE TRANSITIONING TO THE NEXT LIFE

There seem to be some common factors that everyone needs to learn before moving along to the next life. Now perhaps you know about these lessons and learned them early on in this life. Well, so much the better, but if you never had the opportunity, now's your chance.

Letting go is a huge one. When I was visiting my dad in Missouri when he was sick, I asked him why he was still living there when most of his family who loved him was in California. He said, "Because of my *stuff*." From somewhere grace came, and I was able to speak frankly to my dad, something I had never done before. I began, "Well, baby, I'm so sorry to be the one to tell you this. It won't be yours for much longer. So the real question is, where do you want to spend your final days? Here, in Missouri, guarding your *stuff*, or with the people who love you?"

Receiving is equally important, especially for those of us who've been givers in this life. Learning to receive can remain a mystery. It is easy to give but difficult to receive. As it turned out, my dad did come to California, but just for the holidays. While he did keep some control over his life, he learned to receive the love and care his family had to give him.

I suppose if you've been a receiver all your life, then you'll have to learn how to give. Whatever the case is for you—whether you need to learn to give or receive—it's about learning balance.

Trusting is not only about trusting God, but also about yourself. Only you know what is best for you! You can get opinions and advice, but in the end, it's all about you! You decide! Trust that you know what's best for you and trust that God is in control. He sees everything. He knows the hairs on your head. God is ever-present, ever-loving, and with all of us, always.

> *Indeed, the very hairs of your head are all numbered.*
>
> *Do not fear; you are more valuable than the sparrows.*
>
> ~ Luke 12:7

HOW NOT TO *JUST WAIT*

The following tips are given as a guide to help you not "just wait," but to live your life fully, while you're still alive!

> *"Am I going to withdraw from the world, like most people do, or am I going to live? I decided I'm going to live, or at least try to live, the way I want, with dignity, with courage, with humor, and with composure.*

> *There are some mornings when I cry and cry and mourn for myself. Some mornings I'm so angry and bitter. But it doesn't last too long. Then I get up and say, I want to live!"*
>
> ~ Mitch Albom, *Tuesdays with Morrie*

BECOME PROACTIVE WITH YOUR LIFE

Waiting to die is bullshit, (as my dad said during his final days on this earth) if in fact that's what you're doing. By *waiting* I mean simply existing, letting life dictate your days, waiting for someone to call, waiting for someone to come over, waiting for someone to bring you something, to do something for you, to read your mind. Don't get caught in this trap!

What I am suggesting is to take a proactive attitude about your life. Synonyms for the word *proactive* include *upbeat* and *hands on*. To be proactive is to be upbeat and light hearted, and to take a *hands on* approach to living. No matter what anyone says, *nobody* knows when a person is going to be *called home*.

> *If I knew the world was ending tomorrow, I'd still plant my cherry tree today!*
>
> ~ Martin Luther

Ask yourself: How do you want to be remembered? What legacy do you want to leave behind? What would you do if you weren't afraid? How do you want to spend your last days on this earth? Who do you want to be with? How do you want to spend your time? Remember, there are no *shoulds* here!

What do you want to do? It's all about you!

Would you like someone to call you? Call them! You may say, "No, they're busy." But perhaps they would appreciate your making an effort in the relationship. It's not up to you to decide if they're busy or not, it's up to them to tell you if they're too busy for a chat. I would expect they would appreciate a call as much as you would. Maybe they don't know what to say! Would you like someone to stop by for tea? Invite them over. No one is interested in a relationship that is one-sided. Make the effort. Take a drive. If you can't drive or don't feel comfortable driving any longer, let someone drive you! Pretend you're being chauffeured! Then say, "Please call me Miss Daisy!" (Like the movie, *Driving Miss Daisy*.)

> *He had created a cocoon of human activities, conversation, interaction and affection; and it filled his life like an overflowing soup bowl.*
> ~ Mitch Albom, *Tuesdays with Morrie*

TAKE CARE OF YOURSELF . . . GUILT FREE!

Get your toenails clipped, trim the hair on your ears, nose, eyebrows, and chin! Do things that make you feel fabulous! Honor your body. When it needs rest, give it rest. When I saw my dad the last time in Missouri, I said to him, "You need a haircut." "No, I don't," he replied. "Dad, yes you do! How do you want to be remembered—as an eccentric old man or the man of dignity and class that you are?" (We got his eyebrows, ear, and nose hairs trimmed as well!)

> *Do what feels GREAT . . . Do what you've always wanted to do!*

YOU'RE WORTH IT!

My dad lived in what others may consider a shack (he had grand visions of remodeling), and yet his estate was worth over a million and half dollars when he died. I stayed in a hotel when I came to visit. This was an extravagance in my dad's way of thinking. He didn't have a tub at his house. (Well, he did, but it was full of *stuff*!) When I'd come to town, I'd spend the night at the hotel, complete with beautiful towels and bedding. Now and then I could talk him into coming over for the afternoon and a bath. (He slept in a recliner at his house—no bed.) He made a comment one night about how luxurious the towels and bedding were. He deserved nice things. We all deserve nice things! Maybe the hardest part is to feel like we deserve nice things.

God created man in His own image . . .

~ Genesis 1:27

The first time he stayed the night at the hotel on one of my visits, he used the toilet bowl brush to wash his back! I had to tell him we were going to buy him a back scrubbing brush! He wasn't a toilet bowl!

One evening I couldn't help noticing that his toenails needed trimming, badly! He had diabetes, and so they were thick and long. I wasn't very happy about the idea of doing this, so I said to him, "Dad, they have people to do this professionally!" "Yes and it costs forty-dollars," he complained. "Well," I told him, "*You are worth* forty-dollars!"

Use your money to have others help you! Clean, organize, travel! Do whatever it is that will make your life more pleasant. Pay people to make your life nice and comfortable. It's your money! Saving it for a rainy day? Honey, *this* is the rainy day! Spend it!

You may say, "I don't want to spend any money, I want to save it for my children." You spend it or they will, and it will be more fun for everyone if you do! Spend your last penny on your last day here! There is no need for sacrificing. If you want to leave another something, leave them memories of a fun and joyous you!

Spend your last penny on your last day here!

CHANGE YOUR PERSPECTIVE

Life changes, and you will need to go through the emotions of your life possibly turning out differently than you thought it would. A new perspective could help you to see things for what they really are: a gift, a precious gift of time. Time to say and do the things that you never had the time to do.

I went to visit a ninety-year-old friend of mine in Northern California, and I asked her one morning if there was anything she had always wanted to do. She wanted to go to Oregon to see her sister. "Let's go now!" I suggested. "Oh, I couldn't," she answered. "Why not?" I asked. "What else do you have to do?" She thought about it for about five minutes before declaring," Okay!" We hopped in the car, drove to Oregon, spent the night, and drove back. They had the loveliest time together. It was the last time that she saw her sister.

Change the way you look at things . . . be
open to new possibilities!

LETTING GO

I like to use the analogy of a water skier when I think of not letting go. What happens when you're skiing behind a boat and you fall? If you don't let go of the rope, your arms will be pulled out of their sockets, your bathing suit will be pulled down by the water pressure, and water will go up your nose. You will be dragged until you *do* let go, and if you still won't let go, you will get a pulled hamstring! (First-hand experience here!) How much easier it is to let go when you first fall! If you do, you simply float—assuming you're wearing a life jacket, of course! Let go in the beginning or let go after more pain—the choice is up to you. But don't forget it is one of the three final lessons (letting go, receiving, and trusting) that seem inevitable across the board. So do yourself a favor and begin letting go.

> *Give others an opportunity to grow and find their own personal power.*

Let Go of How You Think Things Should Be

You *should* be able to walk as far as you did when you were younger; you *should* be able to drive, pull weeds, do the wash and the cooking. Let go of how you think things *should be* and say *yes* to how they are. Trust that God is in control and is watching. He hasn't forgotten you. You need not worry. Rest in the fact that the body is meant to slow down; it's part of the process of living; it's part of the process of transitioning.

> *Say YES to how things are, instead of how you think they should be!*

Let Go of Judgments of Yourself/Others

Concentrate on you! It's your turn! Don't worry about others, what they may say or may do. This is your time. Let go of your negative judgment of yourself. If you see a negative thought creeping into your head or hear a negative word coming out of your mouth, stop! And consciously turn it into something positive. Even *just kidding* remarks about you or anyone else are negative. Stop yourself! Say something positive and upbeat. The old saying, "If you can't say something nice, don't say anything at all" needs to be refined. We have to take it to the next level. Find something positive to say. This may not be an easy task. When I was learning to think and live in a positive manner, I had to call my friend regularly to help me turn my thoughts and statements into something positive! It's diligent work, but it's worth it in the end! (p.s. the judgments you place on others are just a reflection of the judgments you place on yourself!)

Be kind to yourself; be kind to others!

Let Go of What You Think Others Should Do or Be

When you're not feeling well or you're aging, it's easy to criticize others, especially if you didn't live your life the way you wanted. It is easy to nitpick the lives of others. If you find yourself thinking, "They're my children, they should _____ " (fill in the blank), stop yourself. Let go of what you think others should be doing.

Before I knew of the full extent of my dad's illness, he used to complain to my sister that I never answered my phone. I told her that I was not available to chat with my dad 24/7. (I liked to be prepared for our conversations.) However, I did call him every weekend when I had the time and energy to talk. She told me that *she* didn't even talk to him that often. Since I wasn't available to him (from his viewpoint) whenever he called, he couldn't see that I called to talk to him each week. If he had only changed what he thought *should* happen, he could have enjoyed the gift as it came.

Take responsibility for your own happiness.

Let Go of Your Expectations

Let go of where you think you *should* be living and what you think you *should* be doing. My Irish friend Martha, who had been moved from her house so it could be remodeled, said to me, "I can't believe that I'm living my final days away from my house." Where you physically are has nothing to do with anything. Simply say *yes* and be happy with what has come your way. It's the attitude that you have in your head that matters. (If you find yourself in a home that cares for the elderly or ill, maybe God needs you there to be an example of a positive attitude for the others!)

Take your great attitude along with you!

Let Go of Your Things; Pass Them Along

There's a sense of finality when we begin to get rid of our things, and then the question arises, "What if it's a false alarm? What if I get better? I won't have anything!" But it's not fair that you leave your stuff, or *rubbish,* as the Irish say, for others to clean up! We are taking nothing with us except our love when we leave this world. Get rid of your stuff! I took care of a lady who had very little left in life. She lived in a rest home and the only real possessions that she had left were her stuffed animals. She wanted to be sure that her stuffed animals would not end up in the hands of children. It doesn't matter what is precious to you—it is probably not as precious to anyone else. Let it go, with your blessings, and trust that it will end up in the hands of who is to be the recipient. You will get to see the joy on their face.

Trust that God is in control of this too.

DO NOT KEEP SECRETS FROM YOUR FAMILY AND FRIENDS . . . TALK ABOUT IT! TALK ABOUT EVERYTHING!

Talk and share with your family and your friends. Talk about everything. Ask questions. Answer questions. You are no longer the parent who needs to *protect* anyone. You are not a friend who needs to keep another from feeling pain. Your willingness to participate in your life until the end is your gift to them.

> *Clear, direct communication! Be Crystal clear!*

HOW I FELT WHEN MY DAD TRIED TO "PROCTECT" ME (BY NOT TELLING ME HE WAS DYING)

My cousin and I made a trip to visit my dad while he was sick. On the day we were leaving for the airport, a man and a woman came to the back door. Startled, I said, "Hello." I noticed the name badges read: HOSPICE. "He's on Hospice?" I blurted out. "Yes he is." I was shocked. I was working for a doctor's office at the time, and I knew what being on Hospice meant. I also knew that my dad wasn't feeling perfect and that he had a home nurse, but that's all any of us knew. At that point, I don't think my dad had even taken ownership of his illness.

With tears in my eyes, I said goodbye and my cousin and I headed for the car. The Chaplain asked if he could speak with us before we left. All I wanted to do was run, but I agreed. He told us, "He wouldn't let us tell any of you kids. He's pretty stubborn, but now that you're here, he's agreed to let me speak with you. Do you know what he's dying from?" he asked. I replied, "I know he's got diabetes and congestive heart failure." "In fact," the Chaplain said, "it's renal failure, and he's not going to go on kidney dialysis. You can call our office and speak with a nurse anytime."

I cannot even begin to tell you the pain and anger I felt, along with the feelings of betrayal and of being shut out of my father's life. I know that he did it out of love, that he thought he was protecting us. He didn't want his children to worry about him, but in his secretiveness he cut himself off from the support of those of us who loved him and cared about him the most.

> *Don't try to protect others; trust they are learning lessons as well.*

ASK FOR WHAT YOU NEED AND WANT

Many of us were raised in a time when you weren't encouraged to ask for what you needed, and especially not for what you wanted. You were considered boastful, arrogant, or selfish if you did. I remember watching old-time movies where the nuns weren't allowed to ask for anything at the dinner table. They had to wait until someone noticed and offered the salt or butter, or anticipated that they might have enjoyed more potatoes! People (including me) were trained to be *mind-readers* (truly a co-dependency issue), which is so unfair to everyone! But it doesn't have to be that way. Others are not responsible for your happiness. Others should not be expected to read your mind.

I remember when I got my first real glimpse of this *mind reading* talent that I had become a master of without even realizing it. My dad came to California for a visit and one evening while we were all watching the television, one of my sons asked his grandpa if he would like some ice cream. My dad said "No." I interrupted, "That means he wants two scoops." My son protested, "But he said no, Mom." "I know," I continued, "but that's not what he *means*. He means he wants two scoops!" That was my first peek into the ability I developed to learn to guess what others need and want.

It's not fair to yourself or others. It's time to ask for what you need and want *guilt free!* Do not expect that others should know what your thoughts are! "Loved ones in my life should call if they love and care about me!" Oh for pity's sake, stop already! You call them! Go for what you want and need—if not now ... when? Be an example of clear, direct communication for others! Model what boundaries and self-care look like. It will truly be a gift to them; a gift that they can use for the rest of their life!

> *Go for what you want and need, if not now ... when?*

TRUST THAT GOD IS IN CONTROL

No matter if you're anxious about a progressing illness or if you're simply getting on in years, trust that everything is in Divine Order. God knows exactly what is happening. When you pray, pray in a way of expansion rather than contraction. Pray from a place of love rather than fear. Sometimes in our prayers we sound like whiny kids, pleading with God to do things our way from our point of view. Don't tell God how to do His job. Let Him do things His way. If you do, you won't be disappointed when things don't turn out the way you think they should, from *your* perspective. Trust that all of our souls are on different paths and each one is being provided with what it needs for its highest good. When parents are praying for their children, young or adult, they usually have a way of telling God what and how they want something done.

The Prayers of the Faithful each week at Mass are loaded with this kind of *begging to God* that I'm referring to. For example, say you want to pray for your child's salvation. You may say something like, "Please help Johnny to remain Catholic." You may even think longer prayers are better, and so you give God a litany of suggestions—the exact plan of how you think it should be carried out! If Johnny leaves the church, you may feel let down or abandoned by God. Be assured that God is answering your prayers, but perhaps in a way you're not expecting. I like to say that God uses the back door! Things usually never come in the way that we expect them to.

Maybe in praying from expansion and love, you could say something like, "Thank you for your love of Johnny. I trust that you know exactly what he needs. Thank you for putting people in his path who will help him to remain close to you!" Now, whatever happens with Johnny, you know that it's part of the journey of his soul, and in the end his relationship with God will be exactly what it is supposed to be without any preconceived notions of yours. You get to take a much-needed rest. Now, simply breathe, *Ahhhhhhhhhh!*

Trust that everything is in Divine Order,
created for your highest good!

SAY YES TO WHAT IS ~ ACCEPTANCE

When my life was being transformed into something new (in other words, my life as I had previously known it was over!), I remember looking up to heaven one day and shaking my finger at God. "Excuse me!" I cried, "Are you paying any attention to what's happening down here?" Certainly He was, and when I learned to say *yes*, knowing that something good was going to come out of all this turmoil, peace followed. I now know that at the end of the rainbow there is, in fact, a pot of gold!

Say that you want to be with your *blood* relatives, and instead God sends you someone who has the time to be with you, but you can't appreciate it because all you can see is that you want your kin around. Breathe in and then breathe out. Don't fight it; just relax. Rest in the fact that you trust that God knows what is happening. Simply say *yes* to what comes your way.

When I was taking care of my ninety-year-old friend, I was kinder to her than anyone from her own family. I didn't have a *history* with her. I did things for her, like wipe her bottom (the way she directed), and other things that *kin* possibly wouldn't do. All she could see is that she wanted to be with her *kinfolk,* and the sad part was, they didn't want to be with her. Because of this, she wasn't fully able to receive the blessings of my presence.

Rest in the fact that God is in control!

GIVE THANKS FOR ALL THINGS

Always say *thank you,* whether or not you understand or are happy with what is happening. I assure you that absolutely everything is being orchestrated for your highest good. It's important to remember that we're talking about the *journey of the soul* here; we're talking about eternity.

Everything is part of a Divine Plan.

FIND THE JOY

Find your happy place. Do not let the *shoulds* be part of your vocabulary ("I should go . . . "). You owe your life to no one! It's yours alone. Live consciously; choose *you* in every moment.

> *Do only the things that bring you joy!*

HAVE A PARTY!

Celebrate your family and friends. Celebrate your life! This quote from *Tuesdays with Morrie* exemplifies something Morrie did in his final days: *"He made some calls, chose a date. And on a cold Sunday afternoon, he was joined in his home by a small group of friends and family for a 'living funeral.' Each of them spoke and paid tribute to my old professor. Some cried, some laughed...Morrie cried and laughed with them. And all the heartfelt things we never get to say to those we love, Morrie said that day . . . "*

> *Celebrate your family and friends.*
> *Celebrate your life!*

MAKE YOUR FUNERAL ARRANGEMENTS

I know, you don't want to think about it or talk about it. If you don't think about it, if you just ignore it, it will just go away . . . right? Wrong. It's not going to go away! We're all on the road home, so you may as well pick the songs, readings, and other things that are meaningful to you in your life. It's another thing you can share with your family, and it will give them the opportunity to know you on a deeper level. It's your funeral. How would you like it to be? What is meaningful to you? Your Spirit will be present at the funeral (if you choose it to be), so you may as well have it your way!

On one of my visits to Missouri to see my father, he announced that he wanted to go to town and meet a guy. When we arrived at the town square diner, the man we were to meet was from the Neptune Society. The meeting was about pre-burial arrangements. I sat and watched my dad take off his belt, turn it over, unzip the hidden zipper, and unfold fifteen one-hundred-dollar bills, which he proudly laid on the table. My dad was taking care of his final arrangements—something I was very grateful for. This transaction was a huge gift to me and would cover the cost of the removal and cremation of his body. My dad didn't want to be buried. He thought it was a waste of money. When I asked him about this, he simply said, "Just throw me to the wind." "Dad," I protested, "while it is your decision how you want to leave this earth, the funeral or memorial is not for you, it's for the ones you leave behind. If you don't mind, I'd like to have a service and bury you with mom." He agreed.

Plan your funeral so others get to see a side of you they possibly did not know!

CHANGE YOUR ATTITUDE

Flexibility is key. Change your attitude, no matter how bleak things look or whatever turn your situation takes. There was a story going around on the internet about this very subject that really resonated with me. It was about a little old lady who had to move to a retirement home. She sat and waited patiently while her room was being prepared for her. The nurse came by to see how she was doing and to tell her her new room would be ready soon. The little lady exclaimed, "I love it!" The puzzled nurse said, "Well, shouldn't you wait until you see it before you decide?" The little lady said, "Loving my new room has nothing to do with how it actually looks, it is simply how I arrange things in my head!" She had mastered the art of flexibility and changing her attitude to accommodate her situation.

If you find you have to leave your home and your familiar surroundings, practice learning to be at home *within yourself,* wherever you are, and not needing your things to define you. God sometimes helps us prepare for the transition by physically taking us away from our earthly things. Sometimes we have to leave our *stuff* behind. Hearses do not come with luggage racks. All that we will be taking with us is our love. It makes leaving the body easier if you have already left your things. Again, your things do not define who you are; you are more than the sum of your stuff. Doesn't giving your precious things to others, while you are able to watch them appreciate you and enjoy them, make some sense?

Bitter or better . . . the choice is up to you!

FIND COMPASSION FOR YOURSELF AND THEN FOR OTHERS

"It's too late, when we die, to admit that we don't see eye to eye." These words from the song "In the Living Years" come to mind when I'm thinking about the end of life. It's okay if we don't see eye to eye. We come from different generations, different life experiences. One person isn't wrong or right. Our journeys, our paths, are about learning lessons, perhaps different lessons. We learn from each other.

Compassion for others comes easier than compassion for ourselves at times. Understanding that all of our souls are on different life journeys helps us to find compassion for everyone. Everyone has the freedom to live their lives according to what is true for them. Everyone has value; everyone has a valid place on the wheel of life. We're all interconnected! We all matter!

We may see things differently. One way is not more valuable than another!

We learn from each other.

LET'S REVIEW

Live, live, live! Life is a banquet and most
poor suckers are starving!

—Auntie Mame

⭐ **Be proactive:** Use the time you have left to truly live!

⭐ **Ask yourself:** How do you want to be remembered? What legacy do you want to leave behind?

⭐ **Take care of yourself:** You're worth spending time, energy, and money on!

⭐ **Get your affairs in order:** Financially, physically, and spiritually.

⭐ **Start liquidating:** It is unfair that you leave your rubbish for others to clean up.

⭐ **Give heirlooms and things to those you intend to:** Give them away now! With love! Enjoy their delight!

⭐ **Change your perspective:** See it for what it is: an opportunity, a gift of time!

⭐ **Don't be a martyr:** Talk about what is happening, what you're feeling. Others need you to share.

⭐ **Ask for what you need and want:** It's not selfish. No one knows what you want or need but you!

⭐ **Don't try to protect others:** It's your gift to them; give them an opportunity to grow.

⭐ **Trust that God is in control:** You get the day off! Don't tell him How to do His job!

⭐ **Acceptance:** Say *yes* to what comes your way!

⭐ **Give thanks for all things:** Whether or not you understand or are happy with what is happening.

⭐ **Change your attitude:** Look on the bright side of your life!

⭐ **Find the joy:** Do only what you can do with joy!

⭐ **Have a party:** Don't wait for a funeral that you won't be *physically* present for! Do it now!

⭐ **Make your funeral arrangements:** Pick the songs, readings, and flowers that have meaning to you.

⭐ **Find compassion for yourself, for others:** We come from different generations; we see differently.

It's not that we fear death,
it's that we fear that we come to the
end of our life and realize that
we never really lived!

-Author Unkown

THE LAST SEASON OF LIFE IS . . .

I was recently reflecting on the fact that after a practice or competition, a marathons runner *cools down*, stretches, walks, and takes it easy. They do all these mild motions to help the body transition back to its *non-performing* mode, its natural state. Well, life is a marathon and we have been performing at full throttle. Now, during this last season, it's the *cool down*.

This last season of life happens by design. It is a time for slowing down and preparation; a time for reflection, a time to explore inwardly. It's a time to discover the soul and to know who you are, who you were created to be. It's also designed for you to spend time with yourself and with God. Taking time for ourselves is something that is more difficult to do while living in the hectic pace of everyday life.

"You're on this earth until you can paint
with all the colors of the wind!"

~ Pocahontas, in *Pocahontas*

WHAT TO EXPECT

While there are many books on what to expect in the dying process, trusting *your* intuition about *your* body is the most important thing you can take with you on your journey. Pay attention to how you're feeling, and what you would like to do, eat, and see. How do you want to spend your time?

⭐ Honor your body; trust that your body knows exactly what to do. If you feel tired, rest; if you feel like sleeping, sleep.

⭐ Get rid of the voices in your head that say *you're not trying hard enough*, or the advice from well-intended people! When my mother was getting ready for her transition, I didn't know anything about this, and I just kept *pushing* her. "You're not trying hard enough, you're not exercising, you're not eating right." I was ruthless! But do realize that if you don't use it, you'll lose it! (Your body and mind!)

⭐ Do only things that bring you JOY!

THE FINAL TRANSTION IN THIS LIFE
Do not be afraid to let go! Death does not exist!

Do not be afraid of death. It does not exist. You have to keep a very open channel, an open mind, no fear and great insight and revelations will come to you. You don't have to do anything except learn to get in touch, in silence, within yourself. Get in touch with your own inner self and learn not to be afraid. One way not to be afraid is to know that Death Does Not Exist. Everything in this life has a positive purpose. Get rid of all negativity; view life as a challenge, a testing ground of your own inner resources and strengths. There are no coincidences.

~ Elisabeth Kübler-Ross

I am absolutely certain of the fact that you will not be alone when the time comes for you to leave your body. I observed this with others as well as with my dad. He knew who had come to greet and escort him to the other side. His eyes lit up when I asked him, "Do you see anyone you know yet, dad?"

Even if there is no one present for you in this physical world (some people prefer to leave when no one is around physically), I assure you that your guardian angel and those you loved and who loved you will be there to help you find the way. Any religious figures that were important to you in this life will be there for you as well!

> *From a scientist's viewpoint, beyond a shadow of a doubt, I can assure you, that at the moment of transition, you are never, ever alone.*
>
> ~ Elisabeth Kübler-Ross

> *Everyone is met by the Heaven of each individual's perception. You will cross over or pass through a bridge, a tunnel, mountain pass, Irish green fields . . . to be met by the Light, a light that is whiter than white. It is extremely bright and the more you approach this Light the more you are embraced by the greatest indescribable, unconditional love you could ever imagine. There are no words for it!*
>
> ~ Betty Eadie

HOW MY DAD'S FINAL TRANSITION TOOK PLACE

Christmas had come and gone, and it was January 4, 2006. My sister and niece were due to come for a visit. I had called the hospice nurse that morning and asked her if she would come to check on my dad because I thought he was getting ready to leave. She came and said, "No, he's got several weeks I would think." I commented, "Well, you don't know my dad, because when he's done, he'll leave!" My sister and niece arrived. My dad was sitting on the side of his bed talking with them. After their conversation he simply said, "Well, let's get this show on the road!"

The next morning, my son and daughter-in-law got my dad up and changed his pajamas. My dad was complaining about how bright the light was in the room. They turned off the lights and asked if it was better. "No, it's very bright, too bright!" They thought something was up. They helped him back to bed, and when my sister and I arrived, my dad was asleep. We let him sleep while we talked. By about two o'clock, I knew it was the day. I called for the hospice nurse to order the orange pain-killing liquid. (Since this was going to be my first *hands-on* experience with the transition, giving him the medicine made me feel better! He didn't want it. In fact, he bit the syringe as I tried to give it to him!)

We sat him up in bed and he wanted to say something. His tongue was thick and he couldn't speak. I just kept touching his face, and my sister and her daughter stroked his arms, letting him hold their hands. I played "Calling All Angels," a song that is dear to me. I continued to ask, "Do you see anyone yet, Pop?" a question I had been asking him for the past several weeks. When his eyes lit up, I knew he had an escort. "Just let go, Pop, follow the Light." And with that, he closed his eyes and he was off! True to my dad's personality, he went out with a bang! Literally! Within five minutes of his leaving, there was a crash of thunder and a bolt of lightning outside the bedroom window. He was safely on his way!

After my experience with my mother's crossing over, I knew the soul needed time for the transition from the body. So I prayed in thanksgiving that my father's body would be left where it was for as long as he needed for his transition. It was about five hours. The funeral people kept apologizing, but I just smiled. I knew it was all in Divine Order.

FINAL WORDS

The day before my dad crossed over into his new life, he sat in his blue rocking chair beside his bed and blurted out, "Waiting to die is bullshit!" I had to laugh, and I answered, "Well, I'll have to agree with you on that one, Pop!"

Having experienced the process of dying with my dad, being with him all the way until his last breath, it certainly did feel like the waiting had no purpose. As I complete this project, I appreciate the fact that the *waiting* is an important part of the *journey of the soul,* and for many it's a key component of the migration to oneness with God and heaven.

As with the anticipation of the birth of a child into this world, *death isn't something to be feared, but something to look forward to!* Our bodies die, but our spirit lives on forever!

Learning to love—love for ourselves, love for others, and loving unconditionally—is essential in this lifetime. We love because we are all interconnected. We love because we are all part of the family of the Creator. While loving is high on the list of items to learn here on earth, there are three other things I've been able to identify that we all have to discover as well: (1) Letting go. Letting go of our stuff, our expectations, our constricted viewpoints. (2) Receiving. Receiving graciously the care, love, encouragement, and anything else another has to give from the heart. The question that arises is, "Can we let ourselves receive?" Then finally, (3) trusting. Not only learning to trust in God, but also finding out that we too are worthy of our own trust.

My hope is that you were able to gain some different points of view to contemplate for yourself, seeing if anything rings true for you. Perhaps my own personal experiences provided a bit of comfort that you're not alone on the journey of your soul. We're all in this together!

> **"Do not believe in anything simply because you have heard it . . .** Do not believe in anything simply because it is spoken and rumored by many. Do not believe in anything simply because it is found written in your religious books. Do not believe in anything merely on the authority of your teachers and elders. Do not believe in traditions because they have been handed down for many generations.

But after observation and analysis, when you find that anything agrees with reason and is conducive to the good and benefit of one and all, then accept it and live up to it.

~ The Buddha

My wish for you is that you will have a new or renewed sense of a loving, merciful, and compassionate Creator who is looking forward to our return to Him/Her once we've completed what it is our soul has come to this earth to learn.

My desire is that you find peace, consolation, and enjoyment all parts of your life's journey, and that you fully live every moment that you're alive!

Life should not be a journey to the grave with the intention of arriving safely in an attractive and well preserved body, but rather to skid in sideways, champagne in one hand, strawberries in the other, body thoroughly used up, totally worn out and screaming . . . WOO HOO . . . What a RIDE!"

~ Indian Larry, The Ryan Clan

And with that, I'll leave you with this last thought to ponder from the movie *Dance of the White Dog:*

"*There are no endings, only discoveries!*"

A TRIBUTE TO MY DAD

GOOD BYE, GOOD LUCK,
GOD BLESS YOU

AND MAY THE GOOD LORD TAKE
A LIKING TO YOU,

CUZ IF HE DOESN'T, YOU KNOW,
NOBODY ELSE WILL . . .

~ Sam Miller

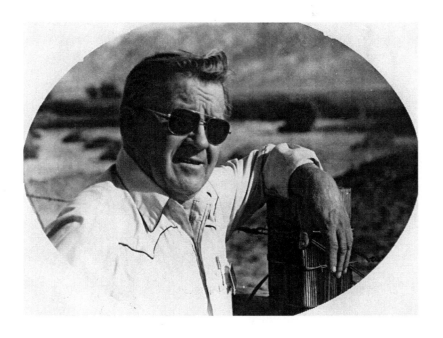

Let me tell you folks who have gathered here today, that I'm a proud and thankful cowboy who has just passed away. I know it's hard but, please don't cry fer I'm now ridin'

Gods trails high up in the sky. I have lived a good life. A cowboy's dream come true. Thank You Lord, fer I'm now ready to ride into eternity. Me, my horse and You.

~ Terry Ike Clanton, "Cowboy's Goodbye"

God, how I hate solemn funerals. When I die, take me into a room and burn me. Then my family and a few good friends should get together, have a few good belts, and talk about the crazy old time we all had together.

~ John Wayne

I've tried to live my life so that my family would love me and my friends respect me. The others can do whatever the hell they please.

~ John Wayne

From my Dad's Memorial Service,
Designed by Brandee Franklin

BIBLIOGRAPHY

Albom, Mitch. *Tuesdays with Morrie.* New York: Random House Publishing, 1997.

D'Arcy, Paula. *A New Set of Eyes.* New York: Crossroads Publishing Company, 2002.

Dass, Ram. *Still Here.* New York: Riverhead Hardcover, 2000.

Dyer, Wayne. *Power of Intention.* Carlsbad, CA: Hay House Publishing, 2005.

Eadie, Betty J. *Embraced By the Light.* New York: Bantam, 1994.

Eadie, Betty J. *The Ripple Effect.* Seattle, WA: Onjinjinkta Publishing, 1999.

Emoto, Masaru. *The Hidden Messages in Water.* Hillsboro, OR: Beyond Words Publishing, 2004.

Karnes, Barbara. *Gone From My Sight: The Dying Experience.* Vancouver, WA: Barbara Karnes Publishing, 1986.

Kempf, Father Joe. *No One Cries the Wrong Way.* Dubuque, IA: Harcourt Religion Publishers, 2003.

Kübler-Ross, Elizabeth. *Life After Death.* Berkley, CA: Celestial Arts, 1991.

Tolle, Eckhart. *The Power of Now.* Novato, CA: New World Library, 1999.

The Holy Bible (New American Standard Edition).

ACKNOWLEDGMENTS

I have a new appreciation for the acknowledgments page in books. It takes many people to make a project come together, whether it's a business idea, an organization, a book, a seminar, or a concert. Whatever it may be, one project takes many heads, hands, and feet working together. As I was reflecting on this, a vision of a centipede came to me. I knew that it meant that one idea to share with others would take the talent of many.

I find this has been true with my project as well. While I think God writes all the books, speaks at all the seminars, etcetera, I have been amazed to watch who He sent with the talents that my project needed just at the right time. I visualized a marathon runner, the coach, the training involved, the pace runner, the people getting the water along the course. For me it's been things others have said, maybe just an insight, a phrase of encouragement, or even a simple smile. When the roadblocks appeared, I looked down the next path and there was someone waiting to cheer me on.

There are many people who won't be publicly recognized for their support, but I would like them to know that I know I couldn't have done it without you! From the plummet of my personal life, to my revival, and every single step of healing that has been inspired and supported along the way, I thank each of you from the bottom of my heart. You have touched my heart and I have gained love, courage, and confidence from your being in my life.

But there are a few key people I'd like to recognize and publicly thank here. It is because of their influence and support that I am still here to share my stories. I'd like to thank my children, Kim, Beca, David, and Jon, for their encouragement and support to move forward with my life. I am forever grateful for the opportunities to learn and grow that are given to me by my family, especially my sister Cathy, not all living in this realm. I continue to feel the presence of their love and encouragement throughout my journey.

Fr. Simon, by your example you showed me what ministering in the spirit was all about, while giving me my first opportunity to work in ministry, and having faith in me to continue my education for the benefit of many. Fr. IK, you helped me understand what was happening when the ground shook in my personal and professional life. You were there to help me stand strong and encouraged me to give others both the opportunity to grow and the space to experience their own strength and power. Thank you my clear-thinking friend.

When my world crashed, Ernie was the first one on the scene with words of encouragement on how to stand back, set goals, and move forward one step at a time. When life as I had previously known it no longer made any sense, Tawni was my mentor and she showed me what self-care and joy was all about. Then Tina picked up the ball and became my cheerleader and cohort. Thanks to Sariah, for her guidance and shamanic gifts, which I believe has to do, in part, with why I am still here in one piece, continuing to grow. Peggy, Geraldine, Bonnie, Jose and Bob, thank you for your support.

To Hannah and her family, for giving me the opportunity to visit Ireland, where I had the space to write this book, find my roots, heal my heart, and connect spiritually with a myriad of support systems, nature, land, sea, and the heavens above, thank you.

Thanks to my friend Teddy, who is always willing to listen and support me in whatever way I need.

Finally, thank you to Bishop Francis Quinn, who believes in me and encourages and supports my ministry work!

And to Barrett, Brooke, and Tabitha, for your expertise in giving life to my experiences.

Thank you to everyone! I love you!

ABOUT THE AUTHOR

Education is not preparation for life;
education is life itself.

~ John Dewey

I am a convert to Catholicism. After becoming a Catholic, I spent the next thirty years volunteering in the Religious Education and Youth Ministry programs. After moving to Northern California, I continued my volunteering and then worked in the Catholic school my children were attending. Later, I began working in administration for the Catholic Church. I had many opportunities to expand my knowledge and strengthen my faith by taking a variety of classes and attending regular retreats. I became the acting principal of Children's Religious Education, then the Director of Religious Education and Coordinator of Junior and Senior High School Youth Ministries. Later I was the director of all church ministries and eventually received a Specialized Certificate in Parish Life and Administration from Loyola University, New Orleans. I loved this work.

However, years later, my life fell apart, and I began to realize that I had been struggling with codependency issues. After several family deaths and the end of a thirty-year marriage through which I now have four adult children, I began searching for the meaning of life for myself. From there, my spiritual gifts had room to emerge.

As I have evolved, I have reinvented myself as an author, inspirational speaker, and workshop/retreat facilitator. In my work, I incorporate many different healing modalities, which include massage and Rising Star Energy Healing. I am a student of spiritual, emotional, and physical healing techniques and am currently based out of Green Valley, Arizona. I refer to my practice as being heart centered. All modalities that I have been drawn to have in the end been around the heart—healing the heart and practicing unconditional love for ourselves, for others, and for the planet.

I believe that humanity is currently moving from a mind-oriented age of knowledge to an era of intuitive and heart-centered knowing. I call this *The Shift,* which I believe will enable us as a society to effectively alter current social structures, values, and modalities of living, to better serve all humanity, the earth, and future generations. I travel internationally, working with individuals, giving lectures, teaching classes, facilitating workshops/retreats, and helping to heal hearts . . . one at a time!

My life experience has prepared me for the work I do today.

~ Pati Hope, Evolve to Live

236

1629

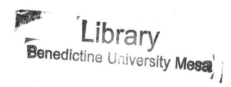

Breinigsville, PA USA
28 December 2010

252309BV00001B/3/P

9 781450 746007